Praise for *The ALF Approach*

"I found the ALF appliance to b_ ____p____i during orthodontic treatment. I highly recommend parents consider the ALF appliance for their children about to embark on orthodontic treatment."

—**Patrick McKeown**, author of *The Oxygen Advantage*

"Dr. Tasha Turzo-Moore shares her in-depth knowledge in a beautifully organized way, using language that appeals to professionals and laypeople alike. I am thrilled that she made such an excellent source available to all of us!"

—**Ljuba Lemke, DMD**, ALF and Wellness Educator

"Combined with osteopathy in the cranial field, the ALF appliance provides safe and gentle healing for a usually very difficult process. This book will take you on a journey that demonstrates these truths and opens a new understanding of the gentleness that holds life together...far more intelligent than Newtonian physics."

—**James Jealous, DO**, author of *An Osteopathic Odyssey*

"Fabulous book! I have worked with patients with an ALF appliance (two of my grandchildren have them!) for almost 40 years and I highly endorse that all dentists, myofunctional therapists, osteopathic physicians and patients with sleep and breathing disorders and craniofacial anomalies read this book! It will change their lives; both personally and professionally."

—**Joy L. Moeller, BS, RDH, OMFT**

"This book is a must-read for any parent considering orthodontics for their child and for any adult with malocclusion or who had orthodontics in the past and now has health problems, even if the problems seem unrelated."

—**Eliott Blackman, DO**

THE ALF APPROACH

Changing the Face of Orthodontics

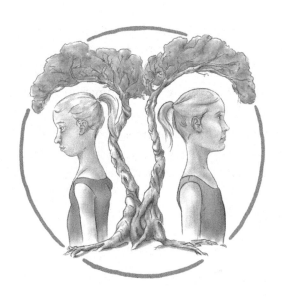

Tasha Turzo-Moore, DO

Printed in the United States of America

ISBN 978-1-7358642-0-4

Published by Transformation Now
www.drtashaturzo.com

This book is dedicated to parents who are striving to create optimal health for their children. May you be inspired and continue to reach for solutions in this challenging era to provide your children with optimal health and well-being. May you have the courage, curiosity, tenacity, and support to meet the needs of the children. They are our future.

Contents

Acknowledgments

With deep gratitude to the people who have inspired this book and supported the process to publication.

I want to thank my editor, Sue Rintoul, for her steadfast and constant support. Thank you for your attention to the details allowing me to focus on the "big picture." I could not have accomplished this without your support.

I want to thank my children, Michaela, Ariela and step (hop-skip-jump) daughter Ana for providing me with the greatest teaching in life. To be your parent has been my greatest joy and challenge. May you know the love that you are and may you move in the world with honor, respect, humility, love and beauty. May your beings transform the world.

I want to thank my beloved husband, Andrew (Rahmat) Moore, MD, whose unyielding love and support is the "wind beneath my wings" and who is the love of my life.

I want to thank my parents, Larry and Jean Edwards, who have dedicated their lives to the transformation of our earth. You have given me the capacities to walk in your footsteps as an educator of transformation. I am forever grateful for your love and support.

I want to thank my illustrator, Adam Knauer, who is a brilliant young budding artist. May your art transform us all.

I want to thank my osteopathic profession and teachers, Drs. Viola Fryman, Eliott Blackman, and James Jealous. Every day I am grateful for your teachings as I have dedicated myself to live, breath, and be of service to the practice and principles of osteopathy. It has truly been an honor to be a part of this family.

I want to thank my dental colleagues and teachers, Drs. Nordstrom and Bronson, who continue to teach me the application of the ALF appliances.

A special thank you to Kathy Winslow, OMFT, and Traci Zimmerman Jones, DO, for their invaluable contribution to this book and their dedication to transformational health.

Last and by no means least, I want to thank my patients for entrusting themselves to my care. You continue to inspire me to "dig deeper" to find the solutions for your health.

You are all my teachers and I am grateful.

Foreword

Darick Nordstrom, DDS

When I graduated from a top-ranked clinical dental school four decades ago, I felt that being awarded top clinician and academic honors would have prepared me to properly provide for my patient's needs. That naive assumption was shattered when our local orthodontist invited me to lunch. He explained that the previous orthodontist had tried too hard to avoid extracting teeth, and failed. He stated, with his authority as an assistant professor and industry consultant, that it just wasn't possible.

I quickly found and joined groups (Crozat, Functional Orthodontics) that were dedicated to avoiding extractions and were more focused on health, and I worked late into the nights to understand the underlying factors that would lead to malocclusions and crowding. I was fortunate to have a gifted pioneer in Oral Myofunctional Therapy come and work together in my office. I was introduced to Osteopathy in the Cranial Field, and found a wonderful practitioner who would work together with my patients. In testing all the orthodontic designs then available, we found that none were truly "cranially compatible"; the Crozat being the least problematic. I took this knowledge, along with that of oral myofunction, and made a design based on the natural principles of growth and development that had been a key part of my quest to understand why patients weren't achieving their full potential.

Working with direct osteopathic feedback, I made refinements based on categorical patient "types." The osteopath then announced that not only were these designs "cranial compatible," but they seemed to have an energy of their own. She described it as if the patient was continuing to receive her treatment after leaving the appointment.

Other osteopaths invited me to work with them and we found that this effect was repeatable and consistent. For the first time, osteopaths were not having to undo the bad effects of orthodontics on their patients. This new form of dental orthopedic treatment was actually augmenting their work; the dentists now becoming key partners in the osteopathic healing paradigm.

As more practitioners learned the technique and began reporting similar results (including the miracles), the word began to spread, leading to the name Alternative Light Force (ALF). The Light Force is based on the principle that the better we understand nature, the less we need to "force" her, in the work to resolve illness and developmental deficiencies.

Dr. Tasha Turzo then took over for the original talented osteopaths who had been part of my early developmental process with ALF. With her energy and talents, we found ways to extend the benefits of this collaborative Osteopathic/ALF interface to the most complex patients. This would drive us even deeper into understanding both "the miracles" and the "why-nots," so that each patient could experience this transformational healing.

Dr. Turzo has a gift for sharing, teaching, and mentoring, and she has been instrumental in training MD, DO, DDS, OMFT/COM, DC, PT, and CST practitioners worldwide in the natural and comprehensive principles behind the miracles of ALF. With her instruction and guidance, you are embarking on a profoundly exciting journey into the understanding of nature's plan for you to achieve your every potential.

James D. Bronson, DDS

There has never been a more appropriate time for this book, *The ALF Approach*, to be published. There is a concentrated search for interdisciplinary treatments to improve our overall health and wellbeing. *The ALF Approach* serves as an introduction into the multifaceted world of the ALF and as an important step into a healthier life!

I have had the honor and privilege to work with Dr. Tasha Turzo starting with my first interdisciplinary ALF case in 2007. Our desire to take the ALF Approach to another level progressed to collaboration on a teaching program that would explain the need and process for advancement of interdisciplinary health treatment with the ALF philosophy, giving birth to the ALF Educational Institute, LLC in 2013. Since that time, we have trained over 120 dentists, osteopaths and myofunctional therapists in the ALF Approach.

Dr. A.T. Still, the father of osteopathy, taught that the body has an inherent ability to heal itself. From the womb of osteopathy the ALF was developed by Dr. Darick Nordstrom. In 1981, utilizing the ALF in movement disorder cases with temporomandibular joint (TMJ) components, Dr. Brendan Stack observed many spontaneous improvements. We have learned to appreciate the remarkable orthodontic advances associated with the ALF appliance, but the physiologic health benefits observed had remained a mystery. As we further understand the worlds of quantum physics, soft matter physics, and biotensegrity, the mysteries of the ALF are becoming clearer.

Physiologically, the ALF acts as a "biomimetic tongue" in normal oral rest posture while also providing subtle neurosensory cellular stimulation and continuous tension support in the cranium, providing for improved balance in the muscles, bones, and fascia of the cranial-mandibular-cervical-respiratory complex. This balance allows the complex systems to free up or borrow energy from the energy drain required to support the previously compromised structure. This energy can then be shunted to a cellular, tissue, or organ system in need of growth or repair. A myriad of far-reaching and sometimes almost magical effects result from this subtle cellular stimulation and congruent biotensegrity balance, such as parasympathetic calming effects, improved breathing, improved sleep, increase in hormone production, improved immune response, less cervical pain, less back pain, less shoulder pain, fewer headaches, improved gait, improved posture, and improved stamina.

Hippocrates said, "Before you heal someone, ask him if he's willing to give up the things that made him sick."

Welcome to a Healthier Happier Life.

Introduction

This book answers questions about the ALF Approach for the DDS/DO/OMFT, as well as for the curious patient/parent. The ALF Approach is an alternative orthodontic process that encompasses a whole-body perspective to changes in the dental occlusion. The body is a dynamic functioning biotensegrity unit that accommodates and grows toward the survival goal of maximizing airway and an upright posture. Any change to one part of the system creates compensation and accommodation to all parts of the body. The dental occlusion is a vital "joint" that not only stabilizes the cranial base but accommodates basic survival functions (swallowing, breathing, chewing, and upright posturing). Therefore, understanding how changes in the dental occlusion affect our health is useful from an integrated perspective. My hope is that this book will provide insight and a potential transformation in how we approach orthodontic dysfunctions in order to optimize health.

Some may wonder, and I would say reasonably so, why an osteopathic physician is teaching, treating, and writing a book about how teeth occlude. Isn't this the realm of orthodontics? Yes it is, and my hope is that the information presented in this book will foster collaboration within the professions of osteopathy, myofunctional therapy, dentistry, and orthodontics to promote an integrated approach to provide patients with optimal treatments. What is the interface between the neuromuscular skeletal system and the position of the teeth? How does the dental occlusion affect the rest of the body? And yes, what causes teeth to be in different positions and why is an osteopathic physician writing a book about tongue function? What is the relevance of tongue function? Don't I just want straight teeth? What are the potential consequences of the traditional orthodontic approach? Hopefully this book will provide answers to these and other questions. My goal for writing this book has been to

1

create a paradigm shift in the approach to traditional orthodontics from a "teeth-focused" perspective to a whole-body and health perspective.

How did I get involved with the ALF appliances and dentistry? The creator of the ALF appliances, Dr. Darick Nordstrom, walked into my office the first Wednesday of the first month of my private practice in 1996. I had taken over a traditional osteopathic practice from a physician who had worked with Dr. Nordstrom for the last several years and thus "inherited" a dentist with my new practice. One of my favorite stories to tell about my adventures with Dr. Nordstrom is how I discovered I would be working with a dentist once a month. I looked at my appointment book and saw that one Wednesday a month was blocked out with the word "Nordstrom" written at the top of the page. I wondered if I had missed an important detail of the purchase of my new practice that meant I was to shop at Nordstrom's one Wednesday a month! As a person who went straight through the educational process from kindergarten to medical internship without breaks, I was thrilled at the idea of just having a day off once a month. I wasn't sure that I wanted to spend the day shopping but was intrigued enough to consider the idea. Who knew that my new practice came with a once-a-month visit from a dentist named Dr. Nordstrom! Over the last 24 years of treating hundreds of patients with the ALF Approach, as well as learning and teaching together, I have written the book as a service to an integrated whole-body approach of the dental occlusion. I believe we are just scratching the surface of what is to come with transformational orthodontics, and I'm excited to continue to learn from my colleagues and patients. We need to keep digging with curiosity as we pursue to understand the big picture of the effects of teeth movement within the whole body.

Why we are facing the face of today. What has happened and what do we do about it?

As this section of the book is titled the "Preface," I find it interesting to compare our human "pre face" and what is now our "current face." The answer is clear. We have sacrificed our airway space (the space behind our tongue and the beginning of our neck) for our ability to move on two legs instead of four. Our mandibles moved backwards as we began to stand upright, limiting airway space. As we began to eat more processed foods and chew less, our mandibles have become less developed and this has resulted in a more "bulldog" facial presentation. Once you begin to recognize the face of compromised function, you will see how prevalent this face is in all cultures. Even more concerning is how an airway-compromised mother develops a fetus with airway-compromised facial features. We are just beginning to investigate this field. The face of a baby born to a mother with a compromised airway is formed and shaped to a less than optimal oxygenated situation. This is a clear expression of "form follows function" and is most likely the reason we as specialists within the neuromuscular skeletal system are seeing an increase in babies born with small mandibles (micrognathia).

Within the last couple of centuries, in a development that was extremely sudden by evolutionary standards, the industrialization of our food supply softened it so much that the human jaw system stopped receiving the same level of functional forces that regulate the growth of the face. The human diet has been softening ever since the use of fire for cooking. It softened further in the transition from hunting to farming. However, it was not until the rapid spread of industrialization in the nineteenth and twentieth centuries that food became so soft it deprived the jaw system of the exercise needed by the jaw muscles to develop properly and stimulate facial growth. Instead of rubbing the lower jawbone against the upper jawbone through the process of forceful chewing, the teeth frequently penetrate the food with a contact, triggering a jaw opening reflex that was designed to protect the teeth by immediately shutting down the activity of the jaw closing muscles. The resulting loss of healthy chewing exercise and the consequential changes in the form and function of the jaw system have significantly altered the pattern of modern human facial growth to produce a number of significant health consequences,[1] which include sleep apnea, diabetes, cardiovascular disease, hypertension, strokes, depression, dementia, and attention deficit disorder (ADD/ADHD).

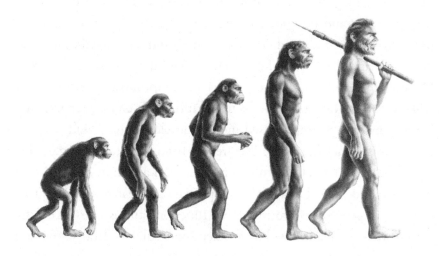

This image shows the diminishing facial growth of humans as we evolved. The face on the far right is shorter from front to back than the other images. This shortens the space behind the tongue, which is the collapsible soft tissue tube called our airway.

Our faces resemble more of a "bulldog" presentation compared to our ancestors, with a diminished maxillary and mandibular forward growth pattern. Dr. Bromage's conclusion was that our modern soft diet is the cause. Our ancestors and their children chewed on bones. Now we feed our children soft foods that are easy to chew, which results in a lack of jaw development. Bone growth is dependent on compressive forces that stimulate osteogenesis (bone growth). If you don't use it, you lose it. We are not chewing on hard substances that stimulate the development of a longer mandibular condyle that results in rotating the mandible forward and increasing the airway space!

It is also interesting to note that sleep-obstructive apnea is increasing. One in four people in the US are diagnosed with mild-to-moderate sleep apnea, and one-third of those have severe sleep apnea. Clearly, our airway is getting smaller. It seems logical to relate this experience with the fact that our faces are flattened (front to back) over time and thus have less airway space, which increases the risk of sleep apnea. This highlights the need to reevaluate our traditional orthodontics approach of moving teeth and the potential narrowing of the airway as a consequence.

There is also a significant rise in the incidence of tongue-ties. Presently, one in three children I see have tongue-ties. Although there is no data documenting the exact increase in incidents at this time, many of my colleagues concur with this increase as their experience.

Why is this? One theory is genetics. The MTHFR gene mutation may be associated with tongue-ties. The basic idea is that patients who have this genetic defect are unable to efficiently detoxify the body, which results in midline defects at birth (example, tongue-tie). There are other conditions associated with this defect, such as recurrent miscarriages, cardiovascular disease, strokes, and cancers. Further investigation is needed in this subject.

Interestingly, malocclusions (crowding and crooked teeth) are also increasing in incidence. Most of the children I see in my practice have crowding of the teeth. Children are supposed to have space between their teeth to hold space for their larger adult teeth. When there are no spaces between teeth, it is considered crowding. We need to identify early signs of airway issues and potential sleep apnea in our children. Crowded teeth in children is not only a sign of a myofunctional dysfunction, but also a risk factor for an airway issue.

Why is there a decrease in facial development over time, an increase in sleep apnea, crowding of the teeth in children, and tongue-ties? Are they all related? Yes, they are all related and have to do with the interplay of our modern diet, environmental toxins, nutrient-poor soil, invasive birth interventions, and loss of the functions that create the face. That's all!

The nutrient richness of our soil is directly related (given no absorption issues) to the microbiome richness of our guts. Poor soil nutrients lead to a poor gut microbiome. As our worldwide farming industry has been exposed to GMO plants and toxic fertilizers, our soil no longer holds the mineral density it used to. For this reason, it is more difficult to raise children on a vegetarian diet. There simply aren't enough nutrients in our veggies to healthily grow our children anymore. They need a nutrient-dense diet to accommodate the challenging world we live in. The book, *Nourishing Traditions*, has an excellent diet for the children of our world today.

This nutrient-poor condition of our lands and foods has also created softer, weaker bone structure. We are now born with a degree of osteopenia (weak bones). We see this in children with changes in the arch structures of the body all the way from a narrow high palate to the collapsing feet arches (pronation). A collapse in structure is occurring. When the palatal bone structure weakens, it bows, creating a high-arched palate.

The cranial bones are also softer and less dense, which can lead to less protection during the birthing process as well as traumatic brain injuries. The combination of increased forces used at birth (vacuum extractions and Pitocin) and a less protective cranium creates a setup for increased cranial strain patterns. Any distortions to the base of the cranium will affect facial growth and development. A baby born with a posterior presentation of the head, also called "sunny side up," experiences compressive forces through the midface due to the obstruction of the mother's pubic symphysis, and could potentially develop an underbite (Class III) facial dysfunction. Any cranial strain pattern to the temporal bone could create a temporomandibular dysfunction as the movement of the mandible is in sync with the movement of the temporal bone.

Curiosity is my favorite mind state. It creates the experience of "I don't know" leading to openness, wonder, and curiosity. Curiosity is an active state of wonder fused with problem solving. This book was written from the state of curiosity, wonder, and problem solving around the etiology, neuromusculoskeletal, and health consequences of malocclusions.

The pandemic of airway compromised individuals calls for a radical paradigm shift in our current orthodontics perspective with its focus on straight teeth and small airways. My goal is for the information in this book to provide an alternative holistic transformative approach to orthodontics and facial growth and development that is based on the need for collaboration within the specialties of dentistry, myofunctional therapy, and osteopathy. The key to understanding the effect of the dental occlusion on the rest of the body lies in essence in the concept of biotensegrity, thixotropy, and the osteopathic principle that the body is one functioning unit, in which structure and function are interrelated and the body has the capacity to heal itself.

The ALF Approach provides a holistic approach to augmenting normal growth and development of the face, aligning the craniocervical junction, "unwinding" cranial strain patterns, and rehabilitating the underlying etiologies for the malocclusion, which always involve the tongue. An integrated approach to orthodontics must include the augmentation of normal facial growth and development, allowing the face to shift forwards. As the face naturally grows forward and downwards, this is called "forward orthodontics." A "backwards orthodontic" approach would move the teeth backward, thus restricting the intra-oral volume compressing the upper cervical vertebrae and limiting room for tongue function.

Transforming traditional orthodontics

Below are three "forward function focused" orthodontists who have experienced a transformation within their profession from the paradigm of "teeth focused" to "whole body health" focused orthodontics. They are pioneering the new pathway as orthodontics becomes a collaborative approach to a potentially transformational healing experience.

Gavin James, BDS, MDS, FDS (Eng), Dip. Orthodont. (Eng, Tor) – Orthodontist

I have been an orthodontist for many years, so when Dr. Turzo invited me to write a chapter in her book I was intrigued. I have long been aware of her work with dental colleagues, in particular with Dr. Darick Nordstrom, and I have used his Advanced Lightwire Functional (ALF) appliance for more than 20 years. As an osteopath, Dr. Turzo works closely with Dr. Nordstrom. I was interested in knowing more about how they used their combination of skills so I asked her to send me the list of her proposed chapter headings. I then attended her two-day webinar and with this experience I was happy to accept her invitation.

The list of titles was confirmation that Dr. Turzo is very familiar with the world of dentistry and understands how osteopathy is an important part of a new orthodontic paradigm. What really caught my attention was that one of her chapters was about biotensegrity. I have now read this chapter and felt an enormous sense of relief at finding a fellow traveler. If you are looking for future developments in orthodontics I suggest you start with Dr. Turzo's book. It provides a firm scientific basis for orthodontists and osteopaths to integrate their skills in a practical way. Better yet, biotensegrity offers a solution to much of the confusion that has troubled the orthodontic specialty for so long.

One of the biggest obstacles to innovation in orthodontic thinking has been the specialty's concentration on the technology of aligning teeth.

The primary concern has been how to correct the malocclusion, not what caused the problem in the first place. This bias is understandable. It is what orthodontists are trained to do. Unfortunately the assumptions on which orthodontists have based their thinking are those of classical mechanics, Newton's most notable contribution to science. These assumptions have stood up very well for several centuries but with the emergence of quantum mechanics it has become clear that live organisms behave differently when compared to non-vital structures.

Obviously the difference has always been there. What has changed is our ability to identify and measure the electromagnetic fields that supply much of the energy keeping the organism alive. The irony is that electromagnetic fields are used for so many other purposes in medicine and dentistry both for diagnostic reasons, such as EMIs, and surgical purposes, such as dissolution of kidney stones to allow them to be passed through the urethra. The major difficulty for an orthodontist is that he or she still thinks in terms of classical common sense mechanics but the body functions in terms of quantum mechanics.

Dr. Turzo's most important insight, in my opinion, has been to recognize this difference and build a treatment approach to solve this apparent discrepancy. As an osteopath, her skills come from manual awareness of differences in body reaction. For an orthodontist, there are several ways to read how the body reacts to the force from orthodontic appliances. In osteopathy the goal is to guide the tissues into a stable position, which is maintained by the overall functioning of the body; that is, it is biocompatible.

In orthodontics, an applied force is intended to move teeth to where the clinician thinks they should be. This difference in objectives is crucial. The orthodontist may well place the teeth where they are prone to relapse. To avoid this possibility he or she may place fixed retainers on the teeth. If a balance within the myofascial tissues has not been achieved previously, these may lock the whole body into a position of excessive stress. Sooner or later the stress will show up somewhere in the system but this reaction will not be seen as connected to earlier orthodontic intervention.

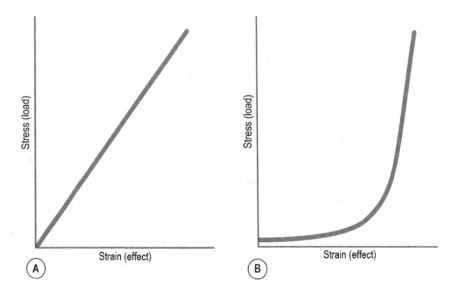

The graphs above show the differences between a non-vital man-made system and a vital organism when reacting to a force. Diagram A represents the non-vital response. The vertical axis indicates the increasing load being applied. The horizontal axis indicates the response to the load. As the load becomes excessive, the reaction of a crane or an engine is likely to be a breakdown of some kind. This has been understood by engineers for more than two centuries. They build safeguards into the machinery well before it reaches a breaking point.

Diagram B is the response of a live organism to a load. The graph starts above the zero point on the vertical axis because a live organism is already under stress. It takes very little increase of load to produce considerable movement of the graph along the horizontal axis. The live organism eventually reacts by becoming more resistant. The more the force increases, the more the organism is prompted to resist the force. At some extreme point, a live organism has to give way but the difference in the reactions of the two types of structure is clear.

It does not take a huge leap of faith for an osteopath to be comfortable with statements like "less is more" or "the whole is greater than the sum of its parts." They experience this scenario every day in their professional lives. They are aware of sources of energy employed by the body as a self-organizing healing system and their techniques are designed to take advantage of this energy. For a conventional orthodontist these statements are well outside their comfort zone. They just don't make sense.

In dental terms a growing number of dentists and osteopaths now understand this contrast in reactions. Dr. Turzo has combined the logic of the ALF philosophy with that of the biotensegrity model. The two concepts are not at odds but complement each other. Several practical conclusions come out of all the theory. It is not meant to ignore the importance of other contributions such as the work of myofunctional therapists. In my opinion a team approach offers the best way to provide answers. Different skills are needed at different points in the continuum from birth to old age. Dr. Turzo's experience in working with such a team has been a great help in expanding the parameters of her thinking, as she readily admits, but there is much more to learn for all of us.

For myself, it has been very rewarding to explore the interesting possibilities for my specialty. I think Dr. Turzo has captured this sense of excitement. Orthodontists have a splendid opportunity to grasp the opportunities opening for them in the health field. Dr. Turzo's book offers them an understanding of how they might start to do so.

Sherry Sami, DDS – Integrative pediatric orthodontist

My evolution as an orthodontist has been driven by an intuitive curiosity that has compelled me to question almost everything I've been taught. As a young resident, I remember looking into the slightly sunken faces of children, all who had four premolar extractions a few years earlier, and wondering whether the long-term effects of our modern interventions did more harm than good. It seemed almost every week I'd see a patient with a new gruesome-looking contraption that was supposed to contain the tongue and correct their dysfunctional swallowing. I don't remember a single case where any of those ghastly appliances made any significant difference for the patient.

It just never made sense to me. Why should someone have to wear a retainer for the rest of their life after orthodontic treatment? That's like telling someone who healed from a broken leg that in order for the bone to stay mended and straight, they'll have to wear a leg brace every night for the rest of their life. Either a therapy works or it doesn't. We either have healing or we don't. It's that simple.

As a pediatric dentist and orthodontist, I was later involved in a craniofacial clinic at UCLA. In spite of my traditional medical education, I'd always known that the body wasn't a collection of mostly isolated parts working in a loose association but rather a singular organism with different aspects all working together in a cohesive interdependence. It was at the craniofacial clinic that I first saw holistic, cohesive healthcare practiced from this perspective. I was amazed to see patients visit each physician and practitioner who afterward met as a team to collaborate on what interventions would be appropriate. Particular attention was paid not only to what therapies would best serve the patient, but the order in which they were administered, and how each intervention was supportive of the others in an effort to achieve the best possible outcome.

Witnessing such a deeply integrative approach to patient care, my curious mind started asking questions again. If our team could provide such comprehensive care to patients, why wasn't the same standard of care available to all patients everywhere? I know physicians consult with and "refer" to each other, but it's not the same thing. Do we really take the time to understand the reasoning of other colleagues on the care team, and how their approach and therapies impact the rest of the plan of care? Do we understand the other parts of the care protocol like we understand our own, and how their interconnected aspects work together to maximize their individual effects?

Those questions were followed up by the words of my beloved teacher from Columbia University, Dr. Melvin Moss, DDS, PhD, ringing in my head: "Don't become a tooth carpenter. It doesn't take much to drill a tooth and fill it. You don't have to get a doctoral degree for it. Become the doctor specializing in the mouth and everything that relates to it. You should be able to look at someone and see how their oral function is affecting their structure without even looking inside the mouth. This is what it means to understand the ontogenetic primacy of function over form." Every day those words remind me to stay focused on the bigger picture of the interconnected and functional nature of the body and not to be focused on form alone.

After residency, I became part of a team of pediatric dentists and orthodontists that collaborated with the Pediatric Medicine Division at the University of California Los Angeles (UCLA) to create a postdoctoral training program in pediatric dentistry with a functional medicine approach called the Children's Health Advocacy Training (CHAT) program. Working closely with pediatric dental and medical professionals, I was inspired to ask more questions. As the answers came, I began to see a profound relationship between the health of the mouth and the rest of the body. Most of these issues were orally-based and determined early in life, such as how breastfeeding affects the development of the mouth and airways.

The life of a pediatric dentist/orthodontist is one of perpetual education, and my next evolution came during a dinner party. My husband, Dr. Habib Sadeghi, is an osteopathic physician and had invited a couple of colleagues over for dinner. As fate would have it, each of those guests invited a couple of friends, and I soon found myself sitting among seven osteopathic physicians and a dentist. During the course of the evening, I was astonished at how much information on functional oral health the dentist was sharing that I'd never heard before. Still, it all made intuitive sense to me and answered many other questions I still had. That dentist was Dr. Darick Nordstrom, the inventor of Advanced Lightwire Functionals (ALF), and his work would change my life.

Shortly after, I started taking classes with him and followed his recommendation on taking courses in cranial osteopathy in order to fully understand the purpose and performance of the appliance he created. In just the first week of my cranial osteopathy training I was overwhelmed, excited, and inspired. I couldn't believe I could actually feel the cranium move and pulsate in what's called primary respiratory rhythm. It made me eager to learn as much as I could as quickly as possible.

It was about this time that I started my own pediatric dentistry and orthodontics practice. In keeping with a functional medicine approach, I made it a priority to place my hands on every patient that came into my office in order to personally examine their oral/cranial function. From this point forward, I had abandoned the traditional orthodontics theory of straightening teeth for aesthetic purposes without any consideration of the other twenty bones in the cranium that are all interconnected like pieces of a puzzle. It just didn't resonate with me anymore. That's when my journey of holistic care that considers body, form, function, emotions, pregnancy and birth experience, generational or personal trauma, nutrition, sleep patterns, medications, parents' health, organ systems, and more truly began.

It's been twelve years since I've been using ALF and osteopathy as the foundation of my practice. In that time, I've learned so much under the direct supervision of my mentor, Dr. Nordstrom, who made regular visits to my office. Many talented osteopathic physicians and teachers later became friends, such as Dr. Tasha Turzo, who was instrumental in helping me understand the relationship between what I do and the rest of the body. All my further education in child development, myofunctional therapy, spiritual psychology with a concentration in consciousness, health and healing, occupational therapy, breathing re-education, sensory integration, and more kept confirming the genius behind the ALF appliance, principles, and design.

It would be a mistake to assume that the ALF is just another orthodontic appliance to expand and make space. To me, the ALF is an orthopedic "invitation" that encourages the body to assume what osteopathic professionals call a midline. By coaxing the tongue, swallowing mechanism, and cranial position to align with the rest of the body, an extraordinary healing power is activated. As the body realigns itself from the top down, the teeth straighten as a natural byproduct of this organic reorganization. When other parts of the body are redirected to assume their natural position through facilitation, not force, the teeth follow suit and the result is a beautiful smile as if the challenge that caused the misalignment had never occurred.

I find it interesting that when I go on my humanitarian trips to remote areas in Guatemala and Honduras, crowded teeth and malocclusion are not the norm in children. While I have seen a few children with collapsed arches and crowded teeth because of early extractions, they are rare exceptions. Crowded teeth and malocclusion among children in the U.S. runs as high as 80% and is considered the norm now. Unfortunately as is the case with traditional medicine much of the time, only the symptom (crowding) of the real problem is addressed rather than looking at the whole person and finding the cause.

I am beyond excited that Dr. Turzo has created such an engaging and informative book about the ALF because I truly believe the ALF journey is a life-changing experience if conducted the right way. Her book also fills a vital need for more resources to train practitioners in the proper usage of the ALF and the furthering of its potential in practice as envisioned by its genius inventor.

Barry Raphael, DMD – Pediatric orthodontist

I was very happy for the first 27 years of my career as a specialist in orthodontics when I first read an article by Dr. German Ramirez who said that "Soft Tissue Dysfunction is the cause of malocclusion" (crooked teeth). It was a concept that a minority of orthodontists had understood even as far back as the late 1800s when orthodontics was just getting started but had never become part of mainstream orthodontic thinking. It is not taught in most modern orthodontic residency programs, and thus, has been largely forgotten by the specialty at large. But for me, curiosity and research led to a new understanding and as of 2020, some 12 years later, I now see orthodontics in a very different way.

In this first chapter, I will give you a sampling of these changes in concept as a way of introducing you to ALF orthodontics and all it has to offer. I'll tell you about what I was taught in school and what I now know to be true.

What I was taught: Malocclusion is the problem and braces are the solution.

Even before I went to orthodontic school, I knew this to be true. In fact, this is the general conception of orthodontics among the public. Everyone who wants straight teeth knows they need braces or aligners. Many parents consider straightening their children's teeth a natural obligation of raising children. They may even carry a sense of guilt that their children's crooked teeth are their "fault" because the assumption is that crooked teeth are inherited from the parents. Even, most orthodontists who know there are many factors that go into the outcome of crooked teeth will say things like, "Yes, you get your teeth from your mother and your jaws from your father and the mismatch creates the crookedness."

Well, did you know that just 400-500 years ago crooked teeth (malocclusion) were a relatively rare phenomenon? While pre-industrial humans had a 3-5% incidence of malocclusion, today as many of 75-80% of children do. No wonder it is now seen as so "normal" to have crooked teeth.

Since it takes tens of thousands of years for a single gene in the human genome to change, genetics cannot be the explanation. Instead, "epigenetics," i.e. how the environment changes gene expression, is more at play here, especially since our environment and culture have changed so drastically in a short period of time.

It is a myth that there are genes for crooked teeth. It has been well documented that when a society moves from their long-standing ancestral diet (usually consisting of whole foods that require lots of chewing to ingest) to a modern, industrial diet (that consists of processed foods that include sugar and artificial ingredients), dental problems such as decay, gum disease, and, yes, malocclusion show up in the very next generation of offspring. And a generation after that, the metabolic disorders that are also now so common as to be thought of as normal - such as heart disease, diabetes, and obesity - begin to show up in the following generations and worsen with each generation in frequency, intensity, and shamefully, at earlier ages of onset.

I will connect the dots for you between food, culture, and chronic disease for you shortly, but let's just say that...

What I now know: Malocclusion is a symptom of a chronic imbalance in the human body.

What I was taught: Genetics is the etiology of malocclusion.

Now that we know that genetics is not the cause of malocclusion, what is? The question implies that we have to find an underlying reason other than the common myth of genetics. In fact, we now know that there are layers of causes that lead up to malocclusion in a tangled web of factors that may differ for each individual. In defining the root cause, we often have to peel the layers of causality like the peeling of an onion.

The reason teeth come in crooked is simply that the jaw bones that contain them have not grown to their full genetic potential and so are not big enough to accommodate the full complement of 32 adult teeth. As teeth erupt into place, they vie for this inadequate space, following a path of least resistance. Hence, they will come in crowded, rotated, slanted, or just out of place.

The upper jaw (maxilla) is particularly apt to undergrow for a variety of reasons. One factor is that this bone requires guidance from the natural positioning of the tongue resting up against the palate (which is the underside of the bone). The tongue acts as a scaffold from which the palate takes its shape. When the tongue has a habit of lying low, as it does with mouth breathing or tongue-tie, the bone takes a different shape, literally collapsing down and inward over the tongue, creating that high-arched palate that is so often seen. With this configuration, teeth don't stand a chance of coming in straight.

Often, with a low tongue posture comes improper tongue function. Swallowing, for instance, is properly done with the tongue also high up against the palate. But many people swallow with their tongue low or forward or in between the teeth. When the tongue has difficulty with the swallow, habits that recruit other facial muscles to help the tongue out are adopted as compensations. These active facial muscles (lips, chin, cheeks, and neck) can put pressure on the teeth and cram them into insufficient space in several common patterns. While many orthodontists think that these patterns are significant, the truth is that they all come from a common etiology.

What I now know: Soft tissue dysfunction is the etiology of malocclusion.

What I was taught: The shape of your face is a personal characteristic.

Orthodontists are known for their anthropomorphic measurements of models of the teeth and x-rays of the face. These "cephalometric" measurements have been studied since the 1940's when the use of x-ray became widely available in dental offices. These measurements have been used to describe different patterns of facial shapes. Terms like "brachyfacial," "dolichofacial," "high-angle," and variations of Angle's classification have been used to not only classify a person's face but to also help guide treatment planning.

One of the assumptions made in using cephalometrics is that the shape of a patient's face is the shape that this person was destined to have; an expression of their genetic birthright. It is true that children do look like their parents to a greater or lesser degree and so there is a degree of gene expression in our face. It is also true, though, that the shape our face ultimately takes can be highly influenced by epigenetic factors as previously explained.

Distortions in the growth of the jaws not only affects the appearance of the face and the eruption of the teeth, but it also affects the shape of the air passages through the nose and throat. If these passages are also smaller than ideal, the very act of breathing can be made more difficult. And since taking the next breath is the most important thing we do moment to moment, a whole new layer of behavioral compensations has to be adopted to keep breathing at an even keel.

The subject of breathing compensations and side-effects goes beyond this current writing, but suffice it to say that when we struggle to breathe, it is a tremendous stress on the body as a whole.

What I now know: The shape of the face can be a risk factor for disease and dysfunction.

What I was taught: The sutures of the bones fuse after puberty.

In dental school, we are taught cranial osteology on dried – and now on plastic – skulls where all the bones seem to be inextricably fused together. The assumption is that all 22 bones of the skull, with the exception of the moveable lower jaw – are bound together so tightly that once fused their growth or position can no longer be altered or influenced.

Doctors of Osteopathy, on the other hand, have been taught that the connections between the bones are flexible throughout life, allowing the bones to constantly adjust and adapt to the demands of function. The functions of the head and neck are numerous – breathing, drinking, chewing, swallowing, speaking, hearing, tasting, smelling, seeing, thinking, and protection of the brain – and all pertinent to our survival. Having a "container" for these functions that is adaptable is a considerable advantage as this book will illustrate.

What I now know: The human skull is a flexible and adaptable structure.

The way orthodontics has been taught in the past makes it almost seem as if the teeth are a separate entity from the rest of the body (hence, the specialty) and that it is okay to ignore imbalances that may have caused a malocclusion. But the new way of thinking makes the alignment of the teeth merely a symptom of an imbalance in the head and requires us to address these imbalances as a prerequisite of orthodontics. Now we must address the imbalances first and then match the teeth to a balanced body.

In this book, Dr. Turzo will show us exactly how that is done and how the orthodontist can be of assistance in creating that balance.

CHAPTER 1

What is an ALF Appliance?

The ALF (Alternative Light Force, also called Advanced Lightwire Functional) is a non-traditional orthopedic/orthodontic, osteopathic, and myofunctional-supportive light wire appliance positioned behind the upper and lower teeth. The wire is fitted on the inside of the teeth to provide the least amount of obstruction for the tongue to rest in the palate. A trained ALF dentist will remove the appliances once a month and widen the loops or bend the body wire approximately 0.25 mm. This changes the shape of the ALF appliance. The change in shape of the appliance and the change in slight pressure in the palate recruits the curious tongue to apply pressure to the newly activated areas and thus changes the shape of the palate. Using the principles of osteopathy to guide the activation of the ALF appliance, the maxilla and mandible advance with a three-dimensional intra-oral expansion, promoting changes in the craniofacial cervical complex and tongue function to achieve a stable, permanent change in dental occlusion, posture, airway and neuro-integration. The wires (0.025-0.028 size) are made of yellow Elgiloy metal.

Goals of the ALF

There are multiple goals with the ALF Approach. The most fundamental goal is to restore and rehabilitate the physiological function of the craniofacial cervical complex (head, face, and neck). With this transformation, teeth position also changes. The position of teeth is influenced by a multitude of soft tissue vector forces of the craniofacial cervical complex that occur during swallowing and chewing, the resting tongue posture, and the somatic biomechanics of the entire soma at rest and in motion. These dynamics are explained throughout this book. Tooth position is primarily the result of contractions of the intraoral soft tissue muscle and the extraoral facial muscle. Individual swallow and chewing patterns have a huge influence on where teeth are positioned. Tooth position is also an influence of the position of the upper and lower jaw in relation to the rest of the face.

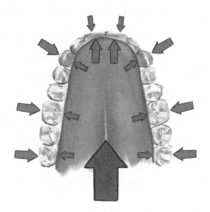

The larger arrow shows the resting position of the tongue in the palate. The outward arrows indicate the vector force of the tongue at rest. These arrows do not indicate the direction of force during a functional swallow but instead the forces of the tongue at rest in the palate. The inward arrows indicate the activation of the facial muscles at rest. The balance between the inward and outward forces of the facial soft tissue and tongue in palate position has a large influence on teeth position. A major contributing factor to teeth position is the direction and force of the tongue and muscles of the face during a swallow.

Another very important and unique goal of the ALF process is to re-establish and integrate the inherent motion of the craniofacial structures. This is fundamentally important as motion is function and function is motion. All the physiological functions in the body are motions that are supported by structures. For example, the flow of a river (function), which creates the riverbed (structure), is like the function of the tongue moving up and back during a normal swallow, creating the structure of a palate. The shape of the riverbed is created by the dynamic flow of water just as the shape and size of the palate is created by the contraction and pressure of the tongue. The subtle motion of the face and a contraction of a functional swallow is what creates the draining of the middle ears and sinuses. Injuries to the craniofacial structure can restrict motion, which can potentially inhibit the "pumping" action the sinuses and middle ear need to drain properly. The ALF is an appliance that augments the inherent craniofacial motion. The wire has a unique balance of strength and flexibility to promote facial growth and development, enhance cranial motion and change teeth position. The ALF was specially designed to be biocompatible with the inherent motion of craniofacial structures. Its augmentation of the motion helps to "unwind" cranial strain patterns, creating more motion and thus health.

The goals of the ALF appliance are to:

- Augment craniofacial motion
- Unwind craniofacial cervical strain patterns
- Provide stability for the cranial base and cervical function
- Encourage neutral tongue-to-palate posturing, which stimulates nasal breathing
- Stimulate normal growth and development of the face

- Reposition teeth and increase airway volume three-dimensionally
- Integrate retained primary reflexes
- Increase glymphatic motion (see Chapter 6)
- Decompress the temporomandibular joint

The initial goals are to restore normal motion and function. Once this has been established, the appliances can be activated to change the position of teeth. Osteopathic principles guide the ALF process in integrating and healing both function and motion, while also transforming the structure. It was not created to be a mechanical device to simply widen the palate; the magic of the appliances lies in their capacity to integrate and restore function *while* the structure of the face is changing.

Development of the ALF

Darick Nordstrom, DDS, is the creator of the ALF. In the 1980s, he began the adventure of creating the ALF appliances. Dr. Nordstrom was working with a "light wire" appliance called the Crozat, which is the predecessor to the ALF appliance. The Crozat is made of a heavier wire than the ALF and has a wire that is placed across the upper palate, which can inhibit tongue function. Also, because of the heavier wires, the inherent craniofacial motion is not activated or augmented and is somewhat impeded.

During the same time, Dr. Nordstrom was introduced to the concepts of cranial osteopathy. He began traveling from his office in Hollister, CA to Santa Cruz, CA to work directly with cranial osteopaths who helped train his hands to feel the subtle cranial motion. Dr. Nordstrom was impressed with the cures of pathologies he saw in the patients being treated by the osteopathic physicians when cranial motion and health was restored. For this reason, he has dedicated himself to creating appliances that increase health by augmenting the inherent craniofacial motion.

During the four-handed treatments, with the osteopathic physician and dentist present together, Dr. Nordstrom used the feedback from the osteopath to make adjustments to the design of the appliances. This was done in order to create a dental appliance that did not create counter compensations throughout the rest of the soma. He also knew that normal tongue function was vital to heal not only malocclusion, but to create optimal airway and overall health.

Dr. Nordstrom's intention was to create a dental appliance that corrected both malocclusion and myofunctional dysfunctions (the major cause of crooked teeth), as well as a cranial-biocompatible appliance that treated cranial strain patterns. He wanted the appliance to restore normal intra-oral function (chewing, swallowing, lip seal posturing, and nasal breathing) and at the same time unwind cranial strain patterns, which he saw as a major underlying cause of malocclusions and many other pathologies. What he created is not simply an orthodontic appliance to widen the palate but more of a health appliance which affects the patient's overall health. Dr. Nordstrom recognized the interplay between neurointegration reflexes, sleep, the dental occlusion, tongue position, and health. He continues to teach and create cutting edge, new horizons concepts and health appliances.

I have been very blessed to be able to treat patients with Dr. Nordstrom and learn from his vast knowledge. We have been treating patients together with four-handed treatments and learning from one another on a monthly basis in Santa Cruz, CA since 1995. The interface between dentistry, osteopathy, myofunctional therapy, and health is vast, and we are still just beginning to explore how to work together in the service of our patients. I am eternally grateful to Dr. Nordstrom for his dedication to perfectionism with perseverance, curiosity, and ingenuity in the creation of the ALF and the team approach to dental and health issues. With deepest respect, thank you Dr. Nordstrom.

Guiding principles of the ALF process

The principles of the ALF Approach *are* the principles of osteopathy. The ALF appliance was created within the womb of osteopathy, as Dr. Nordstrom's intention was to create an osteopathic orthodontic myo-functional appliance. When I teach dentists how to work with the ALF, I tell them they need to understand and embody the principles of osteopathy as these principles will be the guide in adjusting the appliance.

Osteopathic principles

1. *The body is a functional unit.*

We are mostly one drop of fluid from head to toe! It can sometimes be explained that simply. Although we use language to divide the body into separate parts and systems, the whole being including mind, body, spirit, fascia, bones, ligaments, organs, and physiological processes functions as one whole dynamic process, constantly attempting to move towards equilibrium and health. Any change in one system will create a change in others.

There are many examples of the interconnectedness of the human being. Two simple musculoskeletal examples are a twisted ankle affecting the gait, which has consequences for the motion of the hip, pelvis, and back and even potentially the jaw joint. Another is the motion of the shoulder joint, which is intimately connected to the motion of the thoracic, rib, scapular, and cervical system as well as the hip. A compromise to any of the above systems affects the motion of the others. Another example of the unity of the system is seen in the fascia system. The fascia connects all the organs, muscles, bones, ligaments, tendons, lymphatic, venous, arterial and central nervous systems. Any fascial strain affects all the above. The body is a dynamic integrated system that needs to be addressed as a whole functioning unit.

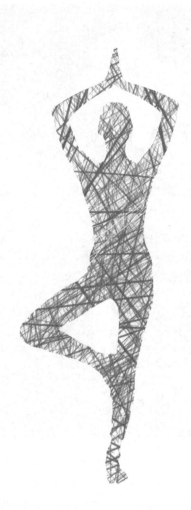

The above picture represents the fascial connections throughout the body. The lines within the images are not anatomical but rather expressive of the interconnection of the attachments that unify the whole body into one functioning unit of motion and function. A subsequent section in this chapter presents the concept of biotensegrity.

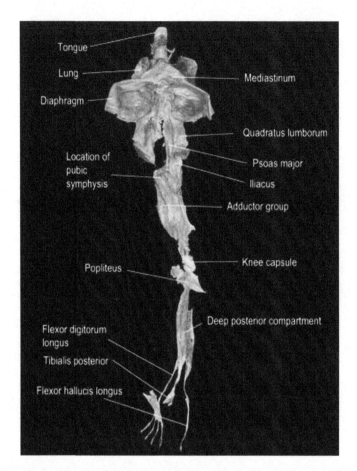

This anatomical dissection depicts the fascial connection from the tongue (top of the picture) down to the toes. Any change in structure or function in the tongue, foot or any anatomical structure in between has an effect on the entire body. This is a clear expression of the body functioning as an integrated unit. The fascia connects the parts into a whole functioning unit.

All the systems of the body provide a check and balance process for each other. For example, the gastrointestinal system is affected by the immune system, which is influenced by the neurological system. In our medical system today we have specialists who are very knowledgeable in one system but do not see the bigger picture of an integrated, whole human being. The pendulum has swung to the extreme of "specialist," but the ALF Approach is the beginning of a collaborative process within professions of sharing knowledge and insights for the benefit of the patient.

The ALF process affects the whole body by integrating and not separating out the dental occlusion from the rest of the body. As the occlusion changes, there are changes in the craniofacial structure and function, as well as every structure and function in the body—even down to the toes!

2. *Structure and function are reciprocally interrelated.*

Consider the formation of a riverbed. The flow of a river (the function) forms the shape of the riverbed (the structure). The shape of the riverbed expresses the history of the flow dynamics of the river. The river and riverbed are interdependent with one another. Just as the development of the palate (mid face) is interdependent with the functions of a correct swallow, correct palatal resting posture of the tongue, and nasal breathing. The structure of the face reflects the functions or dysfunctions which created it. Form follows function.

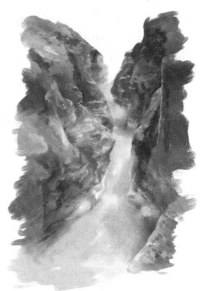

Just as the riverbed tells a story of the flow dynamics of a river, the structure of a face tells the story of the dynamics of the functions of the face. If a myofunctional dysfunction is present, such as an anterior tongue thrust (the tongue moves in a forward motion during swallow as opposed to an up-and-back contraction motion), or the tongue postures behind the lower teeth rather than in the upper palate, then the palate will be underdeveloped and the position of the teeth will be reflected by the movement of the tongue during a dysfunctional swallow pattern. If the palate gets so narrow that the tongue can no longer fit in it, the ALF Approach is needed.

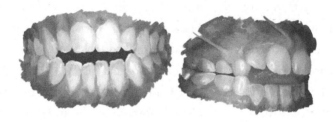

The form (structure) of the dental occlusion expresses the function that created it. Here we see an open bite created by the tongue moving forward during a swallow as opposed to a swallow where the tongue contracts from front to back. The forward moving tongue during swallow pushes the teeth forward and creates an opening. The picture on the left shows the opening in the teeth created by the function of a forward tongue swallow. The picture on the right shows the tongue moving forward during swallow.

The palate (structure) will not maintain its newly expanded form after removal of the ALF if the myofunctional dysfunctions (function) are not corrected. The ALF, osteopathy, and myofunctional therapy rehabilitate the swallow and/or resting lip and tongue posture to change the function. Most orthodontic processes change only the structure and do not address the underlying dysfunctions that create the malocclusion.

For this reason, if a retainer is not worn for the rest of the patient's life there is a 100% rate of relapse with traditional orthodontics because the underlying etiologies were not addressed and therefore the dysfunctions continue.

Because the ALF Approach is based on osteopathic principles, it looks for the structural/functional components and addresses both. The ALF process is an orthodontic process where the patient does not have to wear a dental retainer for the rest of their life. The underlying dysfunctions have to be transformed as the structures of the face are changing. If a somatic or myofunctional dysfunction are not integrated, a relapse of the malocclusion will occur.

3. *The body has the inherent capacity to heal itself.*

Osteopathic physicians approach the patient with the question, "How can I help you help yourself?" We acknowledge that we do not heal the patient but facilitate the healing process by engaging with the tissues/soma to encourage an opening/releasing/unwinding experience. This allows the patient to "let go" into their already present health and perfect being. An osteopathic treatment removes obstacles and restores the body's inherent motion, thus providing the maximum capacity for transformation. Restoring function results in an increase in the flow of arterial, venous blood, cerebral spinal fluid, and lymph, which are the health-giving fluids for all tissues.

This is the same goal of the ALF process. The appliance not only synergistically moves with the cranial bone motions, but also stimulates normal facial growth and development to increase the airway and grow the maxilla/mandibular complex. The ALF helps to restore inherent motion (function), thus removing obstacles and creating potential space for transformation. As is evident from its principles, osteopathy is a humble profession. The sensory information our hands receive allows us to give individualized therapeutic treatments and treatment plans. You, as the patient, are seen and treated as a unique being who is not expected to conform to a "one size fits all" approach.

This is also true for the ALF Approach. The ALF process recognizes the body as a whole functioning unit. The integration of function and structure are the goals. The ALF process helps the individual to realize their greatest potential by removing obstacles and dysfunctions. ALF appliances are uniquely tailored and specifically adjusted for each individual patient. When you look at people's faces that have experienced the ALF processes, their faces "match" the rest of their body.

It's about augmenting motion. Motion is Life and Life is Motion. Osteopathic treatments and ALF adjustments open space and create room for functions to integrate. As this happens, structures are remodeled. This is the outcome of a structure-function inter-relationship.

Why is the type of metal and size of the ALF wire important?

The wire is made of 0.25 to 0.28 yellow Elgiloy metal. ALF appliances can only be made with this size of wire and specific metal. Dr. Nordstrom spent years perfecting the specific material and size of wire to safely augment the cranial motion. He worked with osteopaths to find the perfect combination to activate and stimulate the cranial system, one that was biocompatible with living tissue in motion.

ALF Appliance Basic Anatomy

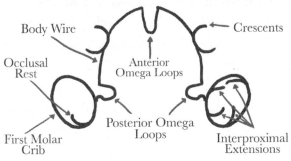

Body Wire

Crescents

Occlusal Rest

Anterior Omega Loops

First Molar Crib

Posterior Omega Loops

Interproximal Extensions

Note: The interproximal extensions are placed on both the right and left molar cribs, as are the occlusal rests.

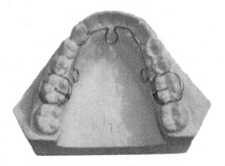

The above image is of an ALF appliance with one anterior and two posterior omega loops, crescents around the canines, and cribs around the first molars with the occlusal rest.

The wire is light and thin but strong enough to stabilize the structures. It bends easily and therefore it's best for the patient to not remove it. There is a "magic" in the structure of the ALF as it has the ability to provide stability and stimulate motion at the same time. It is light enough to allow the subtle inherent motions of the body to breathe without impeding motion while providing the activation needed in the restricted tissues in order to release as well as *move teeth*. It's amazing such a small appliance can do all that!

It is important to also state that the benefits of the ALF happen only with a dentist trained in how to activate and use the ALF. Many dentists and osteopaths using and treating with the ALF have not taken an ALF course. They use the ALF only as a palatal expander but are missing the greater potential healing effects of the ALF process. It is easy to over activate the ALF wires, which inhibits the "magic" of the balance of stability and flexibility of the appliance. The osteopath who has not taken an ALF course does not understand the mechanics of the ALF and thus how to treat the ALF dynamics.

Why and how it works

It's quite simple in theory. The omega loops in the upper appliance attract the curious tongue to rise up and rest in the palate. Once the tongue is up, the lips can rest together and air will travel through the nose and not the mouth. As the lips rest together, the inward pressure of a solid lip seal with tongue pushing upwards within the upper palate begins to align the teeth. Also, as mentioned above, the underlying craniofacial strain patterns will begin to unwind as the tongue applies pressure to the base of the cranium and augments the cranial rhythmic impulse. As this process occurs and osteopathic treatments are incorporated, the alignment between the cranium and cervical bones begins to change, allowing a full body unwinding to occur while teeth are changing position to express the change in function. Remember that the body is one functioning unit, and as the mandibular cranial cervical complex shifts, so do the pelvis and feet.

The tongue is our most potent orthodontic appliance. When the tongue is hand in glove with the palate and there is a "functional" swallow, the palate widens in three dimensions and the space behind the palate (the airway) expands. Because the ALF is always present, it continuously reminds the tongue to return to its normal position. In this way, the ALF is a 24/7 myofunctional appliance as well as a 24/7 osteopathic treatment when activated correctly.

Another very important function of the ALF is to stimulate osteoblastic (bone growth) activity. The contact of the wire stimulates the face to grow and develop new bone. The ALF stimulates facial development by laying down more bone, resulting in a forward growth of the face.

The ALF appliance compared to other orthodontic devices

There are a handful of "light wire" appliances as well as many other orthodontic devices on the market. It can be difficult to choose which appliance would work best for you and/or your family.

Benefits of the ALF

1. The ALF appliance has no obstruction to inhibit potential tongue development of the palate. It recruits the inherent capacity to develop the airway by stimulating the tongue to palatal position.

2. The ALF can rehabilitate myofunctional dysfunctions.

3. The comfort of a light wire allows patients with sensitivities or a very narrow palate to tolerate an orthodontic process.

4. The wires are behind the teeth, making orthodontics an invisible process.

5. The ALF is the only orthodontic appliance that integrates cranial motion with the facial growth and development process. It augments normal cranial motion (if adjusted correctly), thereby helping to resolve cranial strain patterns from birth and head injuries. Other appliances create counter compensation in the cranium and cervical structures as the position of the teeth and jaw joint position are changed, potentially creating more somatic compensatory strain patterns (side effects).

6. The focus of the ALF Approach is the health of the whole body. Most other orthodontic approaches simply focus on the position of the teeth.

7. The ALF Approach is individualized. Each appliance is designed for the individual, and adjustments are made based on the individual's unique oral functions, facial growth patterns, the position of the teeth, and cranial motion. The movement of the cranial structure and face (and whole body) plays a role in adjusting the appliance. There is no generic "one size fits all" adjustment with a turn of a palatal key to expand the palate. Also, the adjustments are not based on creating a face to certain measurements but rather to meet individual needs for transformation and full function.

8. Because the ALF is individualized, your smile and occlusion fit with the rest of the body and personality. Patients who have completed the ALF process typically enjoy an integrated smile, face, cranium, neck, back, pelvis, feet, and gait. When changing the largest occlusion in the body (the dental occlusion), it's best to bring the rest of the body with it in an integrative healing process. This holistic approach to orthodontics is unmatched by any other approach.

9. When the ALF process is complete, there is no need for the use of a lifetime dental retainer. The tongue is the most potent orthodontic influence. Because no other orthodontic appliances address underlying myofunctional and somatic dysfunctions, the myofunctional dysfunction that created the malocclusion in the first place is still present at the end of treatment. This will create a relapse of the facial structure. Other appliances rely only on mechanical activations to create change, while obstructing the tongue, thereby creating a myofunctional dysfunction in the process. The ALF uses our inherent natural physiological process

to develop the palate and face. It allows the craniofacial structures to grow by a natural process and does not "take a face apart" in the process of changing the position of the teeth and widening the palate.

10. The ALF is an oral appliance that develops the palate in three dimensions. Again, this is because the tongue is doing most of the work. The rapid palatal expander develops the palate in only two dimensions, which creates a distorted palate, to say nothing of the unique (and difficult to treat) cranial strain pattern that results from a rapid palatal expander treatment.

11. The ALF is a dental appliance that can be used as early as 3 years old. Early intervention is always the key! Because the ALF simply augments normal growth and development, we are able to halt a facial growth discrepancy and redirect the craniofacial complex back into health with normal functions. With the ALF process in children, changes can be seen within one to two weeks. The child will need less treatment when they are older because their growth discrepancy was redirected at an early age. It is easier to treat children than adults with the ALF. The process is typically shorter with fewer complications because the growth rate is faster in children. The ALF simply augments normal growth and development, so the transformation is faster.

Who could benefit from the ALF Approach?

People with the following conditions:

- Malocclusions/myofunctional dysfunctions
- Traumatic brain injuries
- Birth trauma
- Sleep apnea/airway dysfunctions

- Temporomandibular joint dysfunctions/headaches
- Autism
- Children with the developmental delay spectrum
- Orthodontic trauma
- Ankyloglossia/tongue-tie
- Allergies/asthma
- ADD/ADHD

What grows a face?

The drawing below is a neonatal (within 28 days of birth) skull enlarged to the same size as an adult skull. This depicts the growth difference between a neonatal and an adult craniofacial bony structure.

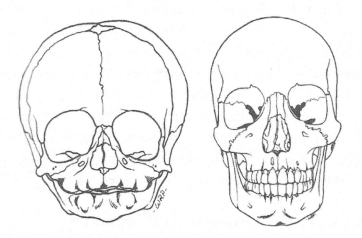

The size of the skull is not that different. In fact 80% of the cranial growth is complete by age two. But there is quite a difference in the shape and size of the face. So what grows a face? It is the function of the face that grows the face. The functions create the structure. Form follows function. Nasal breathing and a tongue to upper palate connection as well as a functional swallow create the mid-face. The newborn is able to breathe, suck, and swallow. These functions lay the foundation of growth stimulation for the maxilla to develop. Chewing creates the size and shape of the mandible. Because a functional swallow creates the maxilla, any myofunctional (swallowing) dysfunctions will create a less than optimal maxilla, which will in turn also affect the growth and development of the mandible.

The neuro-integration of an infant's functional suck and swallow creates the foundation for the resting tongue posture in the palate and its function throughout life. As teeth erupt and the function of chewing begins to coordinate, the mandible is stimulated to grow. The growth of the mandible is influenced not only by which teeth have contact but also the quality of contact of the teeth. The more chewing, the more mandibular development. A soft diet leads to underdeveloped jaws. If the mother has an airway deficiency, sub-optimal oxygenation may result for the fetus, which can affect its mandibular development. These babies are born with an underdeveloped mandible. This makes sense from a "form follows function" paradigm. The baby's structure forms according to the constraints of its physical environment. If there is an environment of sub-optimal oxygenation, the structure that maintains the airway (the mandible) will develop accordingly.

What is an immature swallow and how does a retained immature swallow create malocclusions?

A very important neurodevelopment should occur once the front and back baby teeth have erupted, which usually begins around one year old. A reflex occurs when the new molar teeth contact each other and create a closed container for the tongue. This reflex, which is stimulated by teeth contact, transitions the infantile swallow into an adult swallow, which in turn creates the shape and size of the adult maxilla and mandible.

The infantile swallow is orchestrated by the 7th cranial nerve (the facial nerve). The infantile swallow protrudes the tongue forward to receive nutrients. As the tongue touches the lower lip a reflex is activated to withdraw the tongue back into its cavity. The muscles of swallowing in this infantile reflex are controlled by the facial nerve, which contracts the facial muscles to drive the process of swallowing. The forward and backwards motion of the tongue is the movement of the infantile swallowing pattern. How does this function create the structural form of the mandible? This infantile swallow creates a flat rather than a rounded shape of the top of the jaw bone (mandible). This is also called a flat condylar process.

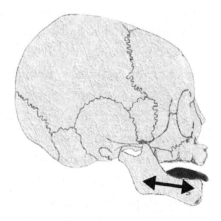

The above image shows the motion of the infantile swallow with a forward and back motion creating a flat mandibular condyle. If the swallowing pattern remains in an infantile (anterior tongue thrust) pattern and the mandibular condyle remains flat in its development, this results in temporomandibular dysfunction.

As the growing child chews, the pattern of swallow should change. Instead of a forward and backward motion of the tongue and mandible motion, the swallow movement is now controlled by the 5th cranial nerve (trigeminal nerve). As the teeth touch, the tongue reflexively moves to rest in the upper palate and the occlusion (teeth touching position) opens to maintain a 1-3 mm space between teeth. This is a neuro-integrated dental occlusion resting posture. Now during swallow, the teeth touch, which brings the tongue to the palate, and then the tongue squeezes up from the tip, middle, and back of the tongue in a wave like motion that propels the food or saliva towards the pharynx (throat). It's also very important to feel the back of the tongue "kick up" with a mature swallow, as this will help to develop the width of the palate.

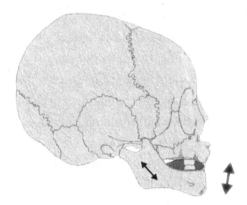

The above image shows the teeth contact stimulating a normal physiological transition to an adult swallow. The mandible is now free to rotate and translate forward to create the normal round shape of the mandibular condyle, which stimulates the temporal bone motion.

The mandible now has a rotational and translational motion, which is also directed by the trigeminal nerve. As the mandible opens and closes, it rotates downward and then moves forward. This motion is what creates the round ball and socket joint of the mandibular condyle. The molar contact with chewing and the forces of chewing are the functions that drive the development of the ramus (the length of the lower jaw). The longer the mandibular ramus (horizontal component of the lower jaw) the more forward the mandible is positioned within the cranium, leaving more room for teeth and the airway in the back of the throat.

A tongue thrust can either be a learned behavior or the result of a tongue-tie. If a learned behavior, it is developed from habits adopted as a child such as digit sucking or the use of a pacifier. A tongue-tie (limited movement of the tongue due to a tight lingual frenulum) results in low tongue posture, thus forcing the tongue to swallow improperly.

Mouth breathing can also result from an immature swallow or tongue thrust (see below); however, the opposite is also true, a tongue thrust can develop from mouth breathing.

So, we can now understand that the transition out of an infantile swallow into a mature swallow is one of the functions that creates the structure of the maxilla and mandible. If this transition does not occur, and there is a retained anterior tongue thrust (immature swallow) where the forward and backward motion of the tongue drags the mandible with it, then the mandibular condyles will form a flat surface. If there is a transition to a mature swallow, where the tongue moves up into the palate with a suction contact and a peristaltic contraction from front to back of the tongue movement with swallow, then the mandibular condyle creates the ball and socket connection of the temporomandibular joint secondary to the rotational and translational movement during a mature swallow. The pattern of muscle contraction of the tongue during a swallow has an effect on the type of movement of the jaw and thus on the developmental shape of the mandible.

There are three parts of an integrated mature swallow: first the tip of the tongue goes up, you bite down to stabilize, and then the tongue contracts with a peristaltic wave squeezing up into the palate. The mandible is free to move slightly forward during a mature swallow. An immature swallow does not allow the mandible's rotational movement as the facial muscles are activated and compress the mandible backwards. The condyle does not develop a rounded shape but remains flat, which reflects the shape of an infant's mandibular condyle form. There is also an increased wear and tear on the disc with a forward and back swallowing pattern and mandibular motion as opposed to the rotational and translational movement of a mature swallow. For this reason, we see temporomandibular dysfunction (TMD) symptoms and structural changes in children and adults with immature swallowing (retained infantile swallow) patterns.

These same TMD symptoms and radiological changes can be seen in children and adults with ankyloglossia (tongue-ties) as the tongue is restricted in its range of motion. This can create the same swallowing patterns as an anterior tongue thrust (or immature swallow).

More is written in this book about TMD in Chapter 6 but what is important to understand here is that the function of swallowing develops first in an infant and then as teeth erupt, chewing integrates. Like all developmental stages, one lays the foundation for the integration and development of the next neurodevelopmental experience. Skipping developmental milestones or leaving one incomplete does not give the next developmental stage a sound foundation. For example, it's very important that babies have a well-coordinated "cross crawl" pattern before they begin to stand. If a baby's leg or foot lags behind with a crawl or the upper body is rotated, this pattern will express itself, even if subtle, in walking, running, and jumping. So, the baby needs to also have a well-integrated suck and swallow before the chewing begins. If the child does not develop a mature swallow pattern, the effects on the mandible will be expressed in symptoms of TMD.

Why would the infantile swallow pattern not integrate to a mature swallow? Prolonged finger or thumb sucking, bottle-feeding, and/or pacifiers will extend the anterior tongue thrust immature swallow. Another very common cause of a dysfunctional swallow pattern is a tongue-tie, also known as ankyloglossia. The tongue has a limited range of motion and thus cannot perform the tongue-to-palate up-and-back sweeping motion of a mature swallow or the lateral motion needed during chewing. Instead the tongue compensates with a limited range of motion and moves forward or laterally (bilateral thrusting) with a swallow, thus stimulating the infantile swallowing patterns and the 7th cranial nerve to help contract the facial muscles, stabilize the jaw and aid in the swallowing process.

Also, the ability of the body to maintain a tongue-to-palate position is a primary reflex that is supposed to integrate starting around 1-2 years of age when the primary molars erupt. The tooth contact stimulates a neuro-integrative process that changes the forward infantile/immature swallow to a mature "up and back" swallow. The neurodevelopment of a child is based on their ability to integrate functions from eye control, sucking and swallow, a cross crawl pattern to standing upright. Primary reflexes are inhibited along the way in development to allow for a balanced upright stance. The transition from an infant suck swallow to an adult suck swallowing pattern is essential in the overall neurological integrative experience as an adult. The ALF appliances can act as a biometric tongue activator in the palate to create a neuro-integration of the infantile swallow. This allows the body to recapitulate a primary reflex that was not integrated and may help other "retained primary reflexes" integrate.

A retained infantile swallow is also associated with asthma, nocturnal asthma, diurnal changes, nocturnal suffocation, apnea, COPD, cough, wheezing, heartburn, chest pain, laryngopharyngeal reflux, laryngitis, ulceration, granuloma, laryngeal carcinoma, chronic hoarseness, pharyngitis, bronchitis, nocturnal choking, and dental diseases.[1-7] As the tongue is the front end of the entire gastrointestinal system, if the movement is aberrant (dysfunctional), that is moving forward instead of a back squeezing and propelling motion, the system as a whole follows the same motion. The forward swallow, which can occur up to 1000 times a day, can create acid reflux (GERD) by pulling acid from the stomach into the esophagus. The infantile swallow creates a negative pressure within the upper gastrointestinal system and reverses the direction of physiological movement of digestion.

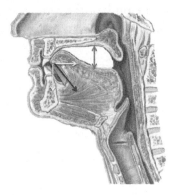 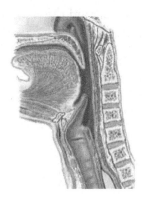

The image above shows a tight frenulum where only the tip of the tongue rests on the palate (behind the upper teeth). The solid bar represents the frenulum; the arrow through the solid bar represents the pull of the frenulum; the arrows to the right and downwards represent the resultant pull of the frenulum in the horizontal and vertical planes; the vertical arrow above the tongue points to one of the eventual effects where the posterior tongue sits low and back, which produces not only sucking, breathing, speech, and TMD problems, but also a narrow posterior palate, as the tongue does not reach the top back of the palate to stimulate growth and development. The image on the right shows the physiological resting position of the tongue with the front, middle, and back parts of the tongue in contact with the palate.

How do I know if my child or I have an immature swallow?

A very basic test for an immature swallow is to insert fingers into the mouth and gently pull the cheeks apart. Holding the checks apart, have the person swallow. You are inhibiting the muscles of the face and the 7th cranial nerve by pulling the cheeks apart. If the person has an infantile swallow, this motion of a swallow will be difficult with the cheeks apart. Spit or bubbles coming out of the front teeth is a sign of an anterior tongue thrust. The tongue is going forward and pushing saliva out from behind the front teeth. The pink of the tongue sticking out from between the teeth is also a sign of an anterior tongue thrust.

During a normal swallow:

- No facial muscles contract or move.

- The head does not move with a swallow. Some people recruit their neck muscles to help them swallow. No head bobbing or nodding with swallowing.

- The head does not move forward with a swallow. This is common with an anterior tongue thrust. The head follows the tongue.

- The eyes do not blink with a swallow. This is another way of recruiting the facial muscle to help with swallowing.

- The person can hold their cheeks apart and swallow with ease.

How to treat an infantile or dysfunctional swallow

It is helpful to identify the etiology of the dysfunctional swallow. If the cause is a traumatic birth with a compression injury to the hypoglossal nerve (see Chapter 3) then off to the cranial osteopath you go. If the immature swallow is from sucking a digit then a myofunctional therapist is needed to get the fingers or thumb out of the mouth. In the end, most if not all myofunctional dysfunctions are helped with myofunctional therapy. Osteopathic treatments are also very helpful to address the soft tissue somatic dysfunctions created by the dysfunctional swallow pattern (aka myofunctional dysfunctions).

A mature/functional swallow augments the cranial motion and facilitates the unwinding of cranial strain patterns

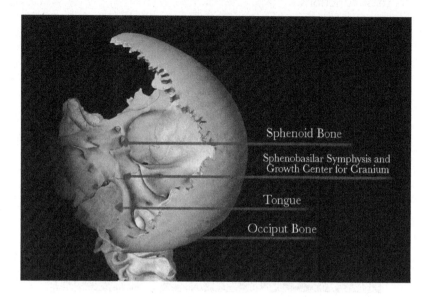

The above image looks down into the cranium to show the connection between the sphenoid and occipital cranial bones, with the tongue lying just below in the oral cavity. The frontal bone, ethmoid, left temporal, and parietal bones have been removed to reveal the sphenobasilar symphysis (SBS), which is a cartilaginous syndesmosis joint that loses its cartilage around 28 years old but retains elasticity and flexibility for motion throughout life. Interestingly, the cranial base, which consists of the ethmoid, sphenoid, and occiput, are developed within embryological cartilage that depends on compressive forces for growth and development.[8] [9]

Swallowing, chewing, and talking are the compressive forces that stimulate the SBS to lay down new occipital and sphenoid bone, thus elongating and growing the cranial base. The length of the cranial base directly influences the forward position of the face. The longer the cranial base, the more forward is the face with a larger airway space. We see here, again, the process of the functional interdependence on the structure. A mature swallow, chewing, and talking are the functions that stimulate the growth of the basicranium, which in turn is a structure that supports these functions.

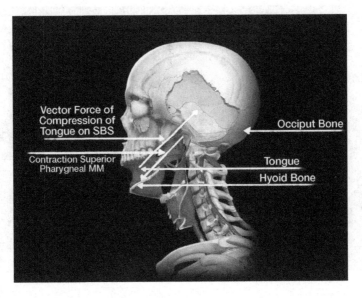

The superior pharyngeal muscle attaches to the occiput just behind the SBS. During a mature/functional swallow, the muscle of the pharynx (superior, middle, and inferior) pulls down specifically on the basiocciput part of the occiput and brings the bone into a backwards nod (cranial flexion). At the same time, the tongue also pushes upwards into the hard and soft palate as the styloglossus muscle that attaches to the styloid process of the temporal bone pulls the back of the tongue up into the hard and soft palate. During a normal swallow, this muscle contracts and pulls the back of the tongue upwards into the cruciate suture of the hard palate and the soft palate. As the back of the tongue compresses the soft tissue, pressure increases into the nasopharyngeal space and into the joint of the cranial base, the sphenobasilar symphysis (SBS).

As the tip of the tongue exerts pressure into the retro incisor spot (the area of the hard palate just behind the two front teeth), the vomer lifts slightly, which transmits motion to the base of the sphenoid just below a vital structure called the sella turcica where the pituitary is housed.

This subtle pressure through the palate to the sphenoid from chewing, swallowing, and talking creates not only a "pumping and draining" action to the middle ear and maxillary sinuses but also into the bowl-like structure (sella turcica). A thin sheath of dural membrane, which is also continuous with the dura throughout the entire cranium, lies over the pituitary stalk. This creates a closed container over the sella turcica that acts as a diaphragm, creating pressure changes that drive the venous and lymphatic drainage of the pituitary. Chapter 6 on glymphatics gives more detail on this subject.

As the tongue pushes up into the base of the sphenoid, the bone flexes subtly down and forwards (called flexion). As described above, the occiput also moves into flexion with swallow as the pharyngeal (swallowing) muscles attach and contract on the occiput. Thus, both the sphenoid and occiput move into flexion as the SBS moves upwards from the compressive forces occurring during a functional swallow. With every functional/ mature swallow, the cranial rhythmic motion is augmented, which not only facilitates the "brain drain" or glymphatic motion but also provides foundational motion to help unwind cranial strain patterns that may have occurred through head injuries or traumatic births. This action of the tongue pressure into the cranium also augments the movement of the cerebral spinal fluids containing vital nutrients to the brain.[10]

The muscle that is specifically associated with contracting the back of the tongue up into the base of the cranium is the styloglossus muscle, which is toned and strengthened through a functional infantile swallow. As this muscle develops its strength through the nursing years, it is then able to bring the back of the tongue into the soft palate with maximum strength to create the pressure changes needed for sinus drainage and cranium motion augmentation. The styloglossus muscle attaches from the intrinsic fibers of the tongue to the styloid process of the temporal bone. Any restrictions, dysfunction, or asymmetrical contraction (between the right and/or left styloglossus muscle) can affect the motion and development of the temporal bone, which most likely will lead to temporomandibular dysfunctions. This is a great example of the interrelationship between the function of the tongue and the structural development of the temporal bone and potential consequential dysfunction of its motion.

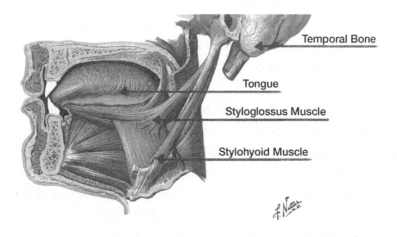

The tongue is directly connected to the temporal bone by the styloglossus muscle. The contraction of this muscle brings the back of the tongue up, compressing into the SBS and widening the back of the palate.

In my experience as a cranial osteopath treating craniofacial dysfunction since 1995, the most difficult craniofacial strain patterns to resolve are with patients who are either tongue-tied and/or have an atypical swallowing pattern in which the front, middle, and back of the tongue do not reach the palate to augment the cranial motion. Many craniofacial strain patterns are symptoms or expressions of myofunctional dysfunctions and malocclusions. Patients with symptoms of atypical swallowing patterns tend to be treatment-dependent with the cranial osteopath because their tongue is not pushing up into the cranial base to decompress the cranium. These patients lack the capacity to heal and unwind cranial trauma without cranial treatments because of the myofunctional dysfunctions. When the patient's swallowing pattern transforms to compress up and back and rests in the upper palate, the cranial strain patterns begin to unwind and are not dependent on cranial treatments.

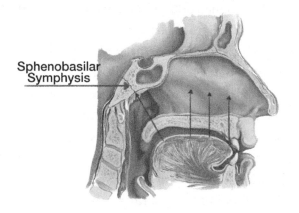

Sphenobasilar
Symphysis

The arrows depict the vector forces of compression the tongue exerts during a mature swallow. The tongue is shaping the upper palate with its contact during times of rest. During a functional swallow, the tongue exerts a pressure through the soft tissue of the upper palate into the space above the soft palate called the nasopharyngeal space. The compressive forces in this area aid in the drainage of the middle ear and sinuses. We see that children with tongue-ties, who lack the tongue range of motion to input a compressive force into the nasopharyngeal, have recurrent middle ear infections. This is commonly missed by cranial osteopaths as most are not looking within the mouth to assess intra-oral function. The tongue's compressive forces are also translated into the most important joint within the cranium, called the sphenobasilar symphysis (SBS). This joint is connected by cartilage. This space continues to have motion throughout life. It is a primary growth center which elongates and grows the base of the cranium bringing the face more forward.

After 28 years, the joint remains pliable for cranial motion, which is essential for venous and lymphatic drainage of the brain. The compressive force into this joint activated by the swallow creates new bone to be deposited on the sphenoid and occiput. The swallow also augments the cranial motion and allows cranial strain patterns to unwind. When an infant has full range of motion of its tongue and the hypoglossal nerve that innervates the tongue is fully functional (Chapter 3), the infants should be able to recover from birth injuries. This is also true as the child grows and experiences head injuries whether they are mild head "bonks" that occur as toddlers learn to walk or severe head injuries with concussion syndrome. Patients who experience traumatic brain injuries will have a more difficult time recovering if the tongue is not able to apply compressive forces into the SBS (also see Chapter 8 TBI). The ALF appliance exerts a force into the palate that not only reminds the tongue of its neutral position but also provides a biometric neural stimulation of the tongue in the roof of the mouth even when the tongue is not in its position in the palate. When there is a myofunctional dysfunction or an immature swallow, the cranium is not stimulated to optimal growth and movement. As a cranial osteopath specializing in craniofacial dysfunction, it is imperative that my palpatory skills are capable of feeling the motion of the cranial base with swallowing. Does the SBS move with the swallow? This is one of the important questions for cranial osteopaths to answer.

The tongue has incredible adaptive capacities. It is not only a sense organ providing tremendous pleasure through taste but it also is a muscle that provides the activities of chewing, swallowing, and speech. It also develops and shapes the midface and plays a large role in the shape and size of the airway. The tongue through its swallowing patterns augments the cranial motion to provide the foundation for optimal lymphatic and venous drainage of the brain to support the brain's health. The compressive forces to the SBS stimulate bone growth for the elongation for the cranial base, which brings the face forwards and thus widens the space in the back of the tongue which is the airway. It can provide stabilization to the jaw joint and will move teeth into a position that optimizes our airway postural capacity.

Here is an interesting piece that was a "wow" to me. A decade ago, Weihenmayer began using the BrainPort, a device that enables him to "see" using his tongue. The BrainPort consists of two parts: the band on his brow supports a tiny video camera; connected to this by a cable is a postage-stamp-size white plastic lollipop, which he holds in his mouth. The camera feed is reduced in resolution to a grid of four hundred gray-scale pixels, transmitted to his tongue via a corresponding grid of four hundred tiny electrodes on the lollipop. Dark pixels provide a strong shock; lighter pixels merely tingle. The resulting vision is a sensation that Weihenmayer describes as "pictures being painted with tiny bubbles."

Neuroscientist Paul Bach-y-Rita hypothesized in the 1960s that "we see with our brains not our eyes." Now, a new device trades on that thinking and aims to partially restore the experience of vision for the blind and visually impaired by relying on the nerves on the tongue's surface to send light signals to the brain.

It remains unclear whether the information is then transferred to the brain's visual cortex, where sight information is normally sent, or to its somatosensory cortex, where touch data from the tongue is interpreted, Wicab neuroscientist Aimee Arnoldussen says. In any case, within 15 minutes of using the device, blind people can begin interpreting spatial information via the BrainPort.

Consequences of ankyloglossia/tongue-tie

Understanding the dynamic and effects of a normal swallowing pattern on facial growth and development helps to explain the vast potential consequences of a tongue with limited range of motion. These consequences include:

- Speech issues

- Malocclusions

- Balance disturbances

- Impeded facial growth and development

- Chronic sinusitis

- Recurrent middle ear infections

- Allergies

- Asthma

- GERD

- Intestinal dysbiosis

- Postural dysfunctions

- Suboptimal cerebral glymphatic and venous drainage

- TMD

- Recurrent gingivitis

What is a functional dental appliance?

A functional dental appliance is an appliance that is essential in restoring normal oral function. There are many appliances advertised on the internet claiming to be a "functional" dental appliance. However, the ALF is the only functional dental appliance that augments and integrates the tongue-to-palate physiological relationship and functions to integrate a mature swallow as well as unwind the craniofacial somatic dysfunction, allowing the entire body to shift to the changes in the dental occlusion. The ALF Approach intention is to bring the entire human being into the transformational dental occlusion process.

The ALF appliances are designed to increase airway, while promoting proper lip seal, nasal breathing, and the tongue's resting posture in the palate. Swallowing, chewing, and breathing are indeed the functions that create a face. So, if an approach shares these goals, then the appliance can be considered a "functional" appliance.

It has become apparent to me that methods of treating malocclusions can be divided into two groups: forward or backward orthodontics. The face naturally grows in a forward and downward movement. Forward orthodontics acknowledges this and enhances this growth pattern. Backward orthodontics is focused on the position of the teeth and alignment without acknowledging the importance of augmenting facial growth and development. Backward approaches typically have wires on the front of teeth, which restrict the forward growth of a face and narrow the airway. The typical facial appearance is a flat midface and small palate with an underdeveloped mandible.

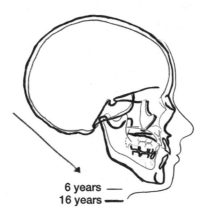

6 years —
16 years —

The above picture shows the forward growth of the face which is driven by the tongue to palate relationship and nasal breathing.

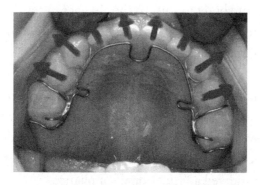

The arrows in the ALF image above indicate the force of growth activation. The palate is expanding from inside to outside and reproducing the activation of the tongue to normal growth and development of the face.

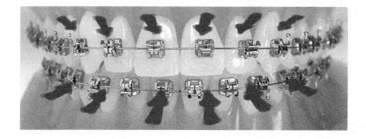

The arrows in this image of the braces indicate a retrusive restrictive growth to the upper and lower jaw, indicating a decrease in intra-oral volume. The direction of movement of the braces depends on the intent of the dentist adjusting the wires and the type of wire used. Some braces do have mild expansive capacities.

Devices based on the forward approach tend to be placed behind the teeth and stimulate forward growth of the maxilla and mandible, creating a more expansive airway space and wider palate.

All "functional" appliances (other than the ALF) have some degree of a palatal barrier that inhibits the normal resting posture of the tongue in the palate. These non-ALF appliances create a myofunctional dysfunction—if the patient didn't need myofunctional therapy before, they will definitely need it after they are removed.

The ALF is the only appliance that rehabilitates myofunctional dysfunction as the teeth are changing position. Why? Because the wire does not cross the palate, which leaves space for the tongue to do the job it was created to do! The tongue is not obstructed and the wires actually attract the curious tongue to posture with the upper palate. When the tongue touches the palate, a reflex for the lips to seal is triggered. Wearing the ALF appliance constantly stimulates and activates this reflex to integrate and restore normal lip seal nasal breathing posture. The keystone to facial growth and development is a competent lip seal and nasal breathing. The ALF Approach restores oral facial function and stimulates the neural integration of primary reflexes throughout the process. Health is restored through the process of stimulating facial growth and development.

The design and force used with other functional appliances results in a disintegration of the craniofacial complex. Strain patterns develop as natural compensation for the over-forceful, over-driving process. Why not use our birth-given, most potent orthodontic appliance called the tongue to naturally do the work it was intended to do? The shape and development of the palate will fit perfectly with the tongue that developed it.

It is also worth noting that the airway space is created by the position and shape of the palate. The ALF process uses the tongue to develop the palate, and the airway is changed in a natural three-dimensional expansion. If you imagine the airway space as a straw, when the front of the straw (maxilla) is pulled forcibly forward, the straw collapses on the sides and is elongated from front to back. Yes, even the space of our airway is created by normal tongue function!

What is a biocompatible appliance?

Biocompatibility means the ability to coexist with living tissues or organisms without causing harm. An appliance that increases and restores function by stimulating forward facial growth and development is not necessarily a biocompatible appliance.

As a physician, I have taken the commitment to "do no harm" to my patients very seriously. If I am not 100% sure that a recommendation will do no harm, I will not recommend it. Dr. Nordstrom shares this commitment and therefore the ALF appliance was created to do no harm. He created an orthodontic appliance that synergizes with the inherent motion of the soma, thus stimulating and augmenting inherent motion and creating the normal growth and development of the face. This allows the whole of the soma to transform along with changes in the dental occlusion.

Other appliances create local change with compensatory changes elsewhere. The heavier the force and the heavier the wires, the more significant are the compensations.

A biocompatible appliance does not need a lifetime retainer to continuously force the occlusion into a shape that is incompatible with the rest of the body. Rehabilitating all myofunctional dysfunctions is an important and inherent part of the ALF process. If there is a myofunctional dysfunction present, there will be a malocclusion relapse. A biocompatible appliance will integrate with the entire soma of the body with seamless biotensegrity without creating non physiological compensatory consequences.

Biotensegrity

Tensegrity is a word coined by Buckminster Fuller based on the words "tension" and "integrity." It refers to a balance of discontinuous compression elements that are connected by continuous tension forces, which allow any system to exist in balance. Biotensegrity refers to this principle as it relates to our bodies, which exist in a delicate balance of tensile and compressive forces that hold all our physical structures in balance. The concepts and principles of biotensegrity (as well as thixotropy, which we will define later) are the key in understanding the effects of osteopathy and the ALF Approach.

The application of the principles of biotensegrity, thixotropy, osteopathy and the dynamics of the ALF Approach serve to augment unwinding and the release of compressed tissue. Restoring flexible tissue helps bring about the essential motion necessary for health. Motion is Life and Life is Motion and Motion is Health.

What is tensegrity?

The integrity of an entire structure is based on its tensional capacity for continuous movement and balance between all the elements. A tensegrity system is one which employs traction (such as with a cable) and the rigidity of other elements (steel, wood, or bamboo) that are capable of acting under the stresses of compression and decompression, in order to provide greater resistance and stability to the overall structure. Tensegrity describes this as "self-tensioning structures composed of rigid structures and cables, with forces of traction and compression, which form an integrated whole."[11]

The principle of tensegrity is one of the many important contributions of the mathematician, artist, and inventor Buckminster Fuller.

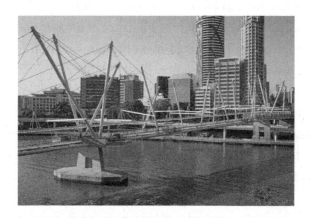

Before Fuller's concept of tensegrity, gravitational and compressive forces were seen as the only stabilizing forces in both architecture and the human body.

The previous model of the human structure with its upright posture of the vertebral column is similar to the concept of buildings that are designed to resist the forces of gravity. In this view the vertebrae are stacked on top of each other and force is passed compressively throughout the spine. This means that all the force passes through the soft disks in between the vertebrae.[12] This model of the body cannot be accurate because the compressive stabilizing forces through the vertebra would not be able to withstand the complexities of locomotion and flexibility of the human structure.

What is biotensegrity?

The integrative model of biotensegrity, developed by Drs. Ingber and Levin in the 1980s, is a perspective that explains the complexities of movement and stability of an interdependent, integrated, complex systems in living organisms. This principle is based on the idea that our bodies are mainly tensegrity structures with an integrated capacity for flexibility and stability with motion as the fulcrum holding the structure together. Yes, motion is the essential component in a biotensegrity system!

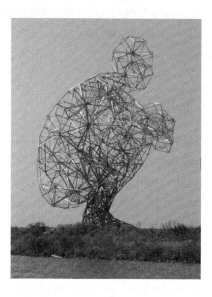

Based on the principles of biotensegrity, our fascial matrix is considered an interconnected tensional network. In this view, our bones are not in direct contact with each other; rather they are floating in the tension structure that is created by our fascial network. Bones and tissues make up a dynamic balance of compression (pushing forces) and tension (pulling forces). Through this global fascial network, any force can influence and create adaptation to any part of the whole, from cells to the entire soma.

In simple terms, the concept of biotensegrity, is a complete shift from the common belief that the bones in the human body are load-bearing structures that work like the framing of a house. Instead, the interconnected structure works biologically with muscles, bones, ligaments, tendons and fascia so that one element strengthens the other creating an interdependent system of movements. Thus, any system of treating the soma of the body needs to incorporate the treatment of the muscles, bones, ligaments, tendons, fascial systems, and organs as one functioning unit of biotensegrity. The craniofacial complex cannot be treated without incorporating the rest of the body as a whole. Any input into the system will create compensatory changes unless it is a biocompatible input that synergizes and augments the motion already present in the living tissues in order to restore the integrity of the entire functioning unit of living tissues.

The importance of motion

Motion is a basic essential component of any tensegrity/biotensegrity structure. The motion necessary in a biotensegrity system is the movement of compression/decompression. This motion provides the flexibility or adaptability needed to be influenced and to influence other tissues in the system. The tissues need to have flexibility and compressibility to be able to accommodate the influences of movements of adjacent tissues. Motion is present in all living systems, and thus restoring inherent physiological motion is the basic goal of an osteopathic physician and the initial goal of the ALF Approach. As motion is restored, there is optimal capacity for the body to heal itself.

The expansion/contraction motion is expressed in all living dynamic systems from the creation of galaxies to the basic unit of life called the cell. Motion is the basis of life and is the essential foundational component needed in a tensegrity system. Our health is dependent on the subtle motion of cellular respiration for vital nutrients to enter the cell and by-products of cellular metabolism (toxins) to exit the cells and enter the lymphatic and venous systems to be filtered and excreted through the lungs, liver, kidneys and skin. This is the process of detoxification.

The cell membrane is made of phospholipids that interlay with one another. The job of our cell membrane is to allow selected nutrients into the cell and allow the waste and toxins (by products of respiration) to leave the cell. It is essential for the cell membrane to be composed of healthy fats, which give flexibility and permeability to the cell wall for passage in and out of the cell in order to maintain optimal cell health.

Consuming higher amounts of omega 6 fats as opposed to omega 3 and 9 fats can result in a more rigid cell wall. This decreased permeability of the cell wall will inhibit the excretion of toxins out of the cell. This is why healthy fats are a vital component for our health as they are the substrates that create the flexibility and fluidity of the cell membrane, allowing toxins to be excreted efficiently.

Another vital compression/decompression movement in the human body is the motion of breathing. The thoracic diaphragm is a musculotendinous structure that transverses the thoracic cage and separates the thoracic cavity from the abdominal cavity. The thoracic diaphragm is attached to the lower six ribs, the sternum and the vertebra body of lumbar vertebra 1 and 2 on the left side and 1-3 on the right side. Openings in the diaphragm allow the esophagus, phrenic and vagus nerves, descending aorta, and inferior vena cava to pass between the thoracic and abdominal cavities.[13]

The movement of this musculotendinous structure is vital for life because the contraction creates negative pressure in the thoracic cavity and positive pressure in the abdominal cavity. The negative thoracic pressure in the thoracic cavity allows vital oxygen to enter the lungs, and the increase in abdominal pressure moves lymphatic and venous fluids against gravity into the lungs, liver, and kidney for detoxification purposes. The thoracic diaphragm also has fascial attachments to not only the heart through the pericardium but also every abdominal organ. The movement of the diagram creates movement in all the organs, which creates the compression/decompression motion that again pumps venous and lymphatic waste products out of the organs and into the system for excretion from the body. Interestingly, the arterial system of our body is held within vessels and innervated by our nervous system as opposed to most of our venous system. Our lymphatic system is not innervated by our nervous system and is completely dependent on contractions of our muscles and fascia systems for movement. This means that our bodies need to have pliability and flexibility of the tissues, especially our rib cage, to have optimal capacity for breathing to create health. The yogis have for centuries claimed that breathing is the key to health and the above explains why this is true.

Integrating and supporting osteopathic principles and treatments

Motion, which is the capacity for stretching and compression is vital for not only the pumping action needed to drive the essential nutrients (blood, venous and lymphatic) into and out of the cells, but also the motion of flexibility and stability is essential to the coherence and integrative capacity for movement of the human body as a whole. The body is one functioning unit. If the entire soma is not treated as "one drop of fluid," an input or force introduced into the tissues or a change in the dental occlusion will create compensatory patterns. Osteopathy and the ALF appliance can release compressions and restrictions in an unwinding process to create a homogeneous whole fluid container, with maximal potential for motion. Once this "neutral" is achieved with osteopathy, myofunctional therapy, and the ALF appliance, the ALF Approach can begin the process of changing (moving teeth with directional intention) the dental occlusion to fit the teeth back together to stabilize the intergrade craniofacial system as well as the entire body.

The ALF Approach is the only orthodontic approach that recognizes the vital importance of integrating the craniofacial movement (especially of the cranial bones) in the treatment of crooked teeth. If the craniofacial motion and cervical motion are not in alignment, and the functional motion of the jaw joint (which is the most important joint and often overlooked) is not integrated back into normal physiological motion, then the new man-made position of the teeth will lock in the craniofacial somatic dysfunction. A malocclusion is the dental expression of the craniofacial cervical dysfunction. When the teeth are forced into a straightened position without the entire craniofacial cervical dysfunction unwinding into a physiological neutral, then the straightened teeth are now locking in compensating craniofacial dysfunction. This is a common and unfortunate situation for many people. Their orthodontically-altered dental occlusion-created compensatory strain patterns are in an already dysfunctional system and now the dental occlusion is preserving the dysfunction. These patients can be difficult to treat osteopathically without the help of the ALF Approach. This is the most common cause of failed somatic release techniques when treating the craniofacial complex. The position of the teeth dictates the position of the maxilla, mandible jaw joint, and cervical vertebrae. It is essential for the tissues to be released and restored to normal physiological motion, with integration of the entire craniofacial complex, before the teeth are repositioned. When an integrated craniofacial complex with jaw joints is moving with freedom, and the intra-oral myofunctions have been restored to normal physiological functions, there will be no need for the use of lifetime or permanent retainers. The underlying etiology of malocclusions will have been addressed!

What is thixotropy?

Thixotropy is the property of a substance of becoming less viscous when subjected to an applied stress.[14] Basically, a thixotropic substance can react as a solid or a liquid, depending on the force introduced to the substance.

Cytoplasm, synovial fluid (found in joints between some bones), ground substance, and mucopolysaccharides in the human body, are all thixotropic.[15]

An example of a thixotropic substance can be created when cornstarch and water are mixed in a 2:1 solution to create a substance known as Oblix, which is analogous to how living tissue responds to stresses. Depending on the force introduced to it, an Oblix solution reacts as a solid or a liquid.

Oblix, like our colloidal tissue, responds with a slow integrative fluid reaction when it is stimulated with a slower fluid-like integrating force. When the solution is agitated the response of the substance is a fluid dynamic with an integrated whole response. If a hard, fast, strong force is inputted into the Oblix solution, the solution reacts as a solid. A solid solution has less movement and does not allow an integrative reaction, but instead has a local reaction. In order for a force to be biocompatible, it has to integrate the input with the whole of the body and all tissues.

The human body, as a biotensegrity structure, requires a slower fluid-like motion to allow the body to remain as a functioning unit and maintain the essential component of motion for health. Rapid, forceful changes in human tissues create local restrictions to motion and result in a dis-integrated state, separating the whole into parts and changing the dynamics of biotensegrity, which threatens the balance of the entire neuromuscular system. This is called somatic dysfunction and is the main underlying cause of pain and neuromuscular dysfunction. Osteopathic treatments engage areas of the body that are hard, compressed and restricted, usually secondary to injury or repetitive use injuries. Through engaging the restricted tissues as a fluid state, these treatments are able to restore physiological motion. The separated hard and compressed tissue is then able to integrate with the whole of the system back into its physiologically fluid state, thus restoring inherent motion and optimal health. The ALF Approach follows the same paradigm of fluidity, biotensegrity, and thixotropy with the goal of integrating and augmenting motion.

Biotensegrity, thixotropy, osteopathy, and the ALF appliance

The unique capacity for flexibility and stability of the ALF appliance, provided by the type and size of the wire, enhance biotensegrity and the thixotropic quality of the craniofacial complex and entire body as a whole. The wire flexes the motion of the cranial bones and augments the inherent motion in the craniofacial complex, allowing the ALF appliance to unwind or restore areas of compressed tissue, i.e. trauma! The ALF appliance also has a compression and decompression, or activating motion, with every swallow, speaking, and chewing experience. These actions augment the motion of the bones and soft tissues of the craniofacial complex increasing motion and thus health. Trauma from compressive forces of the bones and soft tissues compromises the capacity for motion and the vital expansion and compressive forces, "dis ease" results. This can express itself as chronic sinus or middle ear infections in a child. The ALF appliance augments and restores the lost motion and thus re-establishes a neutral state for ongoing breathing movements, which are the fundamental motions for health.

We see the same issues of a loss of functional motion to the temporal bones that is expressed as TMD. The subtle expansion, contraction, motion, and position of the temporal bone is essential to the diffusion of blood, as well as venous and lymphatic flow, to support the health of the disc and the joints' soft tissues. We absolutely cannot treat TMD without the capacity to assess and treat the craniofacial motion that supports the joint position and health (regenerative capacity) of the joint.

The small, individualized, biocompatible activation of the ALF appliance augments motion of the soft tissues as opposed to restricting motion. How the ALF is activated and designed will determine if the appliance is creating a mechanically driven versus a functional fulcrumed process for the patient. The ALF was created with the clear intention of increasing motion as well as restoring and integrating functions that are the etiology of malocclusions and craniofacial dysfunctions. If the ALF dentist is overactivating the appliance, it will become a mechanical device that will create more forceful engagement of the tissues and thus not unwind the restrictions, creating compensatory compressions and strain patterns as a result. The ALF appliance was not created to work as a mechanical device. The ALF appliance is considered to be an "indirect" appliance that augments motion where motion is present. Once the restrictions have been removed, usually with osteopathic treatments, the tissues can be influenced by the ALF without obstacles.

If there is an overwhelming compressive force secondary to trauma or repetitive strain patterns, the process will rely on the osteopathic physician to address and release the compressive forces in the tissue, working with the ALF appliance to integrate and release these compressive forces and restore health. This allows for essential, individual healing to occur. If dentists continue to fall back into their limited, mechanical, Newtonian models taught in dental school for the movement of teeth, compensatory influences will affect the entire craniofacial complex and the position of the dental occlusion will relapse without a lifetime retainer. When the dentist makes individuated and effective adjustments of the ALF, and the decision of where to activate is based on the developing function that is beginning to be integrated, then the dentist is simply following the guide given by functions and leaves no "footprints." This makes the ALF Approach fulcrumed in function as opposed to structure. It's the function that creates our structures, and they are reciprocally interdependent. This is a great challenge for most dentists and requires a large paradigm shift out of an "I'm in charge" mechanical model to one of biotensegrity, thixotropy, non-Newtonian, and osteopathic principles, together with curiosity and observation, in order to determine where, when, and how much to activate the ALF wires. Our more complicated patients are best served with a four-handed team approach, with the osteopathic physician and dentist present together, to problem-solve the more restricted areas in order to apply the right amount of activation to the ALF appliance and augment motion for the individual.

Other orthodontic appliances lack the capacity to augment and restore normal physiological motion of the craniofacial complex. Instead of an unwinding of the compressed injured tissue, these appliances create a forceful, restricted, compensatory reaction to the bones and soft tissue of the face, cranium, mandibular joint, cervical, and on down the body. If the goal is health to the overall system, the means must be to remove obstacles and allow injured parts of the body to integrate into a whole system with optimal motion—in other words, a holistic approach.

CHAPTER 2

Team Approach

The ALF team approach is based on the principles of collaboration: participation, collectivity, transparency, persistence, and mutual professional respect. Following these principles, as we interface within the three professions of dentistry, osteopathy, and orofacial myofunctional therapy, we provide the greatest benefit to the patient for their transformation through the ALF process.

The ALF team consists of an ALF-trained dentist, cranial osteopathic physician, and orofacial myofunctional therapist (OMFT), who have both a professional concern for dental occlusions and the ALF-trained skills to treat craniofacial dysfunctions within their professional scope of practice. We share a common dedication to restore patients' health through working with the ALF appliances, orofacial myofunctional therapy, and osteopathic medicine.

A traditional dentist's formal training is, in general, focused on the oral cavity. While dental education does include the diagnosis and treatment of temporomandibular joint dysfunction, the emphasis is primarily on mandibular repositioning through the use of appliance therapy and surgery. Dental schools do not teach the interrelationship of dental occlusion effects on the cranium, cervical function, swallowing, or overall somatic balance. An integrated educational approach of the dental occlusion with the whole body is not emphasized.

Osteopathic medical education does not include how the dental occlusion affects the neuromuscular skeletal system even though it is the one of the larger joints (by surface area) in the body and is the craniofacial-cervical articulation. The dental occlusion has a direct impact on the motion of the craniofacial cervical complex. Postgraduate courses for the cranial osteopaths in the field of cranial dental dysfunctions are just beginning to emerge, with the challenge of creating a faculty with expertise in this field. Unfortunately, many cranial osteopaths continue to treat the cranial strain patterns that are locked in by the malocclusion. The osteopath is able to release and integrate the cranium but as soon as the patient bites into their malocclusions, the compensatory cranial strain pattern is back, perpetuating the somatic dysfunction previously present. The osteopathic physician must be able to palpate the changes in the cranium created by malocclusions to be able to treat and diagnose cranial strain patterns created by malocclusions. Learning how to diagnose and treat craniofacial cervical dysfunctions created by malocclusions is the first step. My website has information on courses I teach in this field, www.drtashaturzo.com.

The OMFT is trained to diagnose and treat improper tongue rest and functions. How these dysfunctions and compensations impact the cervical vertebrae and cranial motion require a team approach to attain stability. It is important for the OMFT to have the training and understanding of the osteopathic principles and how the ALF works.

I teach dentists, osteopaths, and OMFTs the ALF Approach and the "why behind the wires." In collaboration with an ALF dentist, I teach how to adjust the ALF appliance (see Resources). I encourage the dentist and OMFT to expand their focus to include the whole body instead of the limited oral cavity; and I encourage the osteopathic physician to focus on the oral cavity to understand the intra-oral structure and the functions affecting the cranial and cervical dynamics.

The perspective of each of these professions is extremely valuable as we are working with patients with malocclusions, temporomandibular joint dysfunctions, and craniofacial dysfunctions. It is of utmost importance when working with other professions in a collaborative process to be respectful of each other's knowledge base. It's best for us to approach one another with a sense of curiosity and openness to learning how to best serve the patient.

The players in the ALF team approach are the following:

- ALF-trained dentist (DDS or DMD)
- ALF-trained cranial osteopathic physician (DO)
- ALF-trained orofacial myofunctional therapist (OMFT)

The ALF-trained dentist

The role of the ALF-trained dentist is to assess the occlusions, myofunctional integration, signs and symptoms of airway dysfunctions, sleep health, growth and development of the craniofacial cervical complex, as well as neurological and structural integration. The ALF dentist is trained to ask the important questions about birth, nursing, developmental, sleep, and overall health pertaining to breathing and gut health; as well as physical trauma questions to determine who needs the ALF Approach and when to refer the patient to a cranial osteopathic physician and/or OMFT. The ALF dentist is trained to understand how birth trauma and head injuries affect facial growth, development, and malocclusions.

The dentist will design an individual ALF appliance after taking a mold (or scan) of your teeth. The mold is then sent along with design instructions to an ALF-certified lab to create the appliances. The next step is to insert the upper and lower ALF appliances. They should not be activated on insertion to allow enough time to adjust to the new sensation, usually one month, after which the omega loops are typically adjusted at a rate of 0.25 mm a month. The activations are made by removing the appliance from the mouth, widening the omega loop by 0.25 mm, and then replacing it into the mouth. Which omega loop is activated depends not only on what malocclusion is present but also on the cranial strain patterns present and the movement patterns of the tongue. This is where the dentist needs to be trained to know where and how to activate the appliance.

It is imperative that the ALF dentist understands that the initial phase of activation is simply to keep up with the widening of the palate created by the tongue-to-palate dynamic, which is the driving force for the initial changes. Overly aggressive activation of the ALF will negatively affect cranial motion, as well as flare the teeth if the attempt to change is faster than the maxilla can accommodate. Slow and small activations allow the initial unwinding process to take place. Once the body and the cranial strain patterns are released, a more directed activation and approach can be taken.

My website www.drtashaturzo.com has a list of ALF-trained dentists who have completed the collaborative and integrative ALF training through the ALF Educational Institute, which includes a practical and written exam (see Resources).

The ALF Approach is very different from traditional orthodontics, so having a sound education in adjusting the ALF wires as well as understanding the basic principles of treatment are essential. Patients should be encouraged to ask their dentist about their ALF training and how much experience they have using ALF appliances to make sure they are in competent hands. These days, as the ALF is becoming more popular, it is very common for many dentists to advertise on websites that they provide the ALF, but have NO training in any courses! So, patients, please beware. These dentists are trying to lure you in only to sell you on another dental appliance or use the ALF without any formal training. Become educated and ask the pertinent questions to assess the dentist's ALF experience. Ask what ALF training they have taken and how long they have been using the appliance.

The ALF-trained cranial osteopathic physician

The ALF Approach was developed in accordance with osteopathic principles. Therefore, the practitioner working with the tissues of the body in the ALF process needs to practice within these concepts to be able to integrate the ALF forces. The ALF osteopathic physician needs to have the skills to palpate the influences of the dental occlusion while palpating the cranium. The practitioner needs to be educated and experienced in palpating the subtle motions of the craniofacial complex as well as engaging the patient as a whole integrated fluid complex to ensure that as the occlusion is changing, there is full integration of the changes through all the soma. This makes the difference between a whole, transformative experience versus an isolated mechanical change in the system that inevitably creates counter compensations (strain patterns). Unfortunately, if the osteopathic physician is not treating the body as a whole system, the compensating strains created by heavy wires and forceful appliances will be missed as their perspective is not wide enough to recognize the newly created strain pattern.

What is osteopathy?

Dr. A.T. Still is the founder of osteopathy. He was born in 1828 in Virginia. His father was a Methodist minister and physician. Early in his life, he began an apprenticeship under his father to study medicine and become a physician. Dr. Still became a licensed MD in the state of Missouri and went on to complete additional coursework at the College of Physicians and Surgeons in Kansas City, MO. He also served as a surgeon in the Union Army during the Civil War.

During this time period of the mid 1800s medical treatments were crude, consisting of using small doses of poison as medicine, blood-letting, and what would now be considered barbaric surgeries. Dr. Still's life changed when his four children died of meningitis in 1864. He lost hope in traditional medicine and devoted the next decade of his life to understanding the human body and creating new tools for treating diseases.

Dr. Still was mechanically minded and had a humble, curious nature. He noticed the connection between specific structures and their functions. For example, the structure of a bridge is created in a specific form to accommodate the travel of horse and buggy. He then related this concept to the human body, seeing that bones are formed in a specific design for specific functions. Dysfunctional structures compromise their functions. He began to develop tools (modalities) to treat the human structure to improve health. Soon he was able to cure pathologies like pneumonia by restoring normal rib function, thus allowing the body to restore its maximum lung capacity and oxygen exchange.

His research and clinical observations led him to believe that the musculoskeletal system played a vital role in health and disease. He concluded that the body contained all the elements needed to maintain health. Dr. Still believed that by correcting problems in the body's structure through the use of manual techniques now known as osteopathic manipulative medicine (OMM), the body's ability to heal itself could be greatly improved. He also promoted the idea of preventive medicine and endorsed the philosophy that physicians should focus on treating the whole patient, rather than just the disease. These beliefs formed the basis of a new medical approach, osteopathic medicine. Using this philosophy, Dr. Still opened the first school of osteopathic medicine in Kirksville, MO in 1892. Dr. Still was a supporter of the suffragette movement, with women representing a larger portion of his first class!

He called his new system of medicine "osteopathy" (osteon is Greek for bone), because it was based on anatomy. Dr. Still developed his methods of diagnosis and treatment by relying on the belief that the human being should be treated as a unit. A person cannot get sick in one area of the body without having other areas affected. All body systems operate in unison. He was truly the first holistic physician.

OMM is based on the principle that the human body possesses self-healing/self-regulating mechanisms that are the source of true healing. The focus in treatment, therefore, goes beyond simple spinal alignment, to dealing directly with abnormal body physiology, using an array of direct and indirect techniques. This more holistic healthcare perspective affords the osteopath a broader spectrum of therapeutic options in addition to thrust techniques, there are myofascial release, muscle energy, counterstrain, visceral manipulation, osteopathy in the cranial field, and biodynamics. The osteopath primarily focuses on the functions of the body, which is the health of the system.

The goal is to remove obstacles, augment motion, and restore health. Imagine the body as a river with boulders of varying sizes obstructing the flow. As osteopaths, our hands are trained to dissolve the boulder (restrictions in tissue or fluid) thus allowing fluids to move unobstructed, restoring health.

The following image is a beautiful expression of the human body as a river. Structurally composed of 60% fluid, it follows the principles of biotensegrity and thixotropy; a fluid river analogy expresses what my hands feel during an osteopathic treatment. Boulders within the river (as seen in the right knee in the above image) will change the compressibility and pliability of the local tissue, indicating somatic dysfunction.

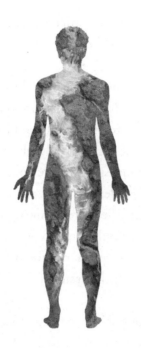

This broader range of diagnostic and therapeutic options allows the osteopathic physician to custom fit their treatment plan to the patient's unique needs, respecting the fact that each of us is not meant to look and function the same way. The goal is not symmetry and alignment as much as full functional motion to all parts of the human being.

What are the differences between an MD and a DO?

Currently, in the United States there are two political bodies that are responsible for providing a medical education and giving a medical degree. The American Osteopathic Association (AOA) regulates a four-year osteopathic medical training and provides the degree of Doctor of Osteopathic Medicine (DO). Presently there are 37 accredited osteopathic medical schools and 57 campuses across the United States. The American Medical Association (AMA) regulates a four-year program for the degree of Medical Doctor. There are 141 accredited MD medical schools in the United States.

After completion of a DO or an MD medical school training program, the doctor must complete a minimum of a one-year internship in the hospital to receive a license to practice medicine. These days most doctors complete at least three to five years of residency to become a specialist in family medicine, internal medicine, surgery, obstetrics and gynecology, and other specialties. Residency programs across the United States accept osteopathic and allopathic physicians into their programs on equal grounds, in fact in 2020 the AOA and AMA's accrediting body the Accreditation Council for the Graduate Medical Education (ACGME) joined into one postgraduate match to place physicians into residencies. Medical schools for DOs and MDs remain separate.

Basically, both medical education systems give the same basic curriculum, except that osteopaths receive education in the diagnosis and treatment of the musculoskeletal system as well as the philosophy and practice of osteopathy. The musculoskeletal system includes the bones, ligaments, tendons, and fascia, as well as the interplay of how these anatomical structures play a part in the overall health and biomechanics of the body. Dr. Still taught his students that the "artery is supreme." He was emphasizing the importance of the dynamic unimpeded movements of the fluids of the body, with blood flow being most important for health. Again, when there is motion in all aspects of the human body, there is health. When there are restrictions, compression, and obstacles to movement, there is less function and overall less health.

Both DOs and MDs have to pass stringent national or state medical board examinations in order to practice medicine. Osteopathic physicians use all the tools available to modern medicine including prescription medication and surgery. DOs, trained in OMM, may use manual techniques to diagnose illness and injury, relieve pain, restore range of motion, and enhance the body's capacity to heal. Unfortunately, there are not many DOs who are practicing OMM as a specialty and what has been termed traditional osteopathy is now considered to be a specialty in osteopathic neuromusculoskeletal medicine (ONMM).

Reflective of the osteopathic philosophy of treating the whole person, many osteopaths serve in the primary care fields: family medicine, general internal medicine, and pediatrics. There is also a long tradition of osteopathic physicians establishing practices in rural and medically underserved areas.

Both American osteopathic physicians (DO) and European osteopaths (OMTh) have studied and trained within osteopathic institutions teaching osteopathic practice and principles. American practitioners are Doctors of Osteopathic Medicine, and European practitioners have a Diploma of Osteopathy. There is, thus, some confusion regarding the difference between US osteopathic physicians and osteopaths trained in other countries. To this day, OMTh's are not physicians. They practice as a therapist of osteopathy. Their training focuses solely on the musculoskeletal system, and they are not licensed to prescribe medications or perform surgeries. They are trained in the practice of osteopathic manipulative techniques and not medicine.

Conversely, US-trained osteopathic physicians practice the entire scope of modern medicine, bringing a patient-centered, holistic, hands-on approach to diagnosing and treating illness and injury. American osteopathic physicians can practice any specialty, prescribe drugs, perform surgeries, and practice medicine anywhere in the United States. American DOs have full medical practice rights throughout the United States and in 44 countries abroad. They bring the additional benefits of osteopathic manipulative techniques to diagnose and treat patients. However, confusing as it may be, most DOs in America do not practice manual osteopathic medicine. Practicing osteopathically with hands-on manual treatments has now become a specialty within medicine. Some of these osteopathic residency programs are now accepting MDs into the specialty of ONMM, which is the current name for the board certification of a specialist within osteopathic medicine.

Osteopathic manipulative medicine as a specialty

An osteopathic physician can specialize in ONMM for which Board Certification became available in 1990. Certification for Osteopathic Cranial Manipulative Medicine is provided by The Osteopathic Cranial Academy, which is currently held by approximately 150 physicians nationwide. All osteopathic physicians are required to attend and document 40 hours of continuing medical education credits each year. For specialists in ONMM, 50 hours of continuing advanced training is required.

What is cranial osteopathy?

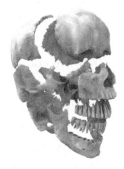

A disarticulated skull and face

William Garner Sutherland, DO, was a student of Dr. Still's at the American School of Osteopathy in 1899. It was during this time that he noticed that the shape of the sutures between the cranial bones were beveled like the gills of a fish, indicating that they were moved by a respiratory, or breathing, mechanism. He spent the next 30 years testing this theory by experiments on his own body. What he discovered was a previously unknown level of physiologic function within the living human being, which he named the primary respiratory mechanism (PRM). This is now commonly known as the "cranial rhythm." The proper function of this PRM is of fundamental importance, not only in the physiology of growth and development of the face, but also in the physiology of healing.

Dr. Sutherland described different aspects of the PRM, including the motility of the neural tube, the mobility of the cranial membranes and bones, and a core link between the cranium and sacrum that coordinates their motion. He identified the fluctuation of the cerebrospinal fluid as the first and most fundamental principle of this mechanism.

Sharon Gustowski, DO, published a thorough literature search from 2010 to 2019, demystifying cranial osteopathy. There is consensus within the medical communities that cranial bones have growth and developmental motion until around 28 years old, and that the sphenobasilar symphysis is a cartilaginous joint in the middle of the head and is a growth center for the cranium. The areas of controversy revolve around sutural closure after 28 years old. To date, the motion of the cranium is 0.29 microns to 1.5 millimeters.[1][2][3] There are many studies investigating this physiology and hopefully the research will continue.[4-18] From the paradigm perspective of biotensegrity and osteopathy, the human body is one functioning unit of motion. This includes the cranial bones, which are held together with fascia interwoven through the interdigitating sutures that fuse with the external scalp, as well as the dural membranes within the cranium. This fascial system has several functions, including acting as a shock absorber during a head injury. The spaces between the cranial bones are filled with fascia that are compressible when cranial bones are impacted from trauma. This compressibility of the tissues protects the brain from further impact. This is the same mechanism by which the brain is protected during the birthing process.

Those doctors who utilize osteopathic cranial manipulative medicine (OCMM) have many hours of additional training in the various functions of the cranium and its relationship to all the anatomic and physiologic systems in the living human system. This specialized training allows the osteopathic physician to diagnose and treat disorders and diseases in ways that are unique to this method of osteopathic diagnosis and treatment.

What is the difference between an osteopathic physician and a chiropractor?

The primary differences between an osteopathic physician and a chiropractor are their levels of training. A chiropractor is not a fully licensed medical physician and is not required to have hospital or medical training. The extent of chiropractic practice is defined by statute as "including the diagnosing and locating of misaligned or displaced vertebrae and, through manual manipulation and adjustment of the spine and other skeletal structures, treating disorders of the human body. The practice of chiropractic does not include the use of drugs or surgery, or the practice of osteopathy, obstetrics, or any other branch of medicine."

History tells an interesting story about the connection between chiropractic and osteopathy. Daniel David Palmer is the founder of chiropractic. He was a grocer who turned magnetic healer and opened an office of magnetic healing in Davenport, Iowa in 1886. When DD Palmer was still a grocer, he saw Dr. Still as a patient in Kirksville, Missouri. Dr. Still used a "thrust" technique, which is one of the many modalities used in osteopathy to treat somatic dysfunction, and Palmer's ailment was cured. Palmer later took that one osteopathic technique and created chiropractic. He opened the first college of chiropractors in 1897. Dr. Still started the first school of osteopathic medicine in 1892.

Comparison of Osteopathic Physicians, Allopathic Physicians, and Chiropractors

	Doctor of Osteopathic Medicine (DO)	*Medical Doctor (MD)*	*Doctor of Chiropractic (DO)*
Undergraduate Training	4 year degree	Same	90 hours college credit Some require degree
Graduate Training	4 year Osteopathic Medical degree (DO)	4 year Medical degree (MD)	4 year Chiropractic degree (DC)
Post Graduate Training	1 year internship 2-8 years residency depending upon the specialty	Same Same	None None
Licensure/ Scope of Practice	Fully licensed to practice the complete spectrum of medical and surgical specialties in all 50 states	Same	Licensed to practice Chiropractic Manipulation
Prescribe Medications	Yes	Same	No
Manual Medicine Training	100-800 hours depending on the school's curriculum	None	Over 500 hours

The chiropractic perspective is primarily focused on the alignment of the spine, which influences the relationship between the spinal column and the nervous system. The chiropractor endeavors to influence the physiological functions of all the organs and systems within the body by changing the position of the spinal vertebrae. The chiropractor is focused on alignment of the structure of the spine and symmetry. In general, most chiropractors use a high force, thrust technique to change the position of the vertebrae although some are trained in gentler methods. Most chiropractors also recommend repetitive adjustment on a weekly basis. The osteopath's goal is to provide freedom in unrestricted motion and function to optimize the health of the system.

There is a significant concern and potential detrimental consequence of repetitive thrust adjustments. The ligaments and tendons around the vertebra are the stabilizers of the spine. With the repeated shearing forces that occur with thrust, there can be a long term compromise to the integrity of the ligaments and tendons, thus affecting the stability of the vertebra and spinal column. The only successful cure that I have found in treating long-term chiropractic high force adjustments that create hypermobility syndrome is prolotherapy/platelet-rich plasma (PRP) injections, which help to regenerate the ligamentous structures.

What is the difference between cranial osteopathy and craniosacral therapy?

Comparison of Osteopathic Physicians and Craniosacral Therapists

	Doctor of Osteopathic Medicine (DO)	*Craniosacral Therapist (CST)*
Graduate Training	4 years of medical school.	Physical therapists, chiropractors or massage therapists. No healthcare license is needed.
Post Grad Training	1-8 years residency training depending on specialty. 140 hours post graduate training with a minimum of three years of practice, a 40-hour basic cranial course, a rigorous written, oral and practical exam is required for Cranial Osteopathy certification.	One 4-day course is necessary to begin practicing. Two 4-day courses are required for certification.
Licensure/ Scope of Practice	Fully licensed to practice the complete spectrum of medical and surgical specialties in all 50 states.	No state or federal licensure and no governing body.
Professional Organizations	In 1939, William G. Sutherland, DO, a student of Dr. Still's, introduced Cranial Osteopathy, the application of osteopathic principles to the cranium.	John Upledger, DO, introduced CST in 1983 teaching to non-physicians. No credit is given to Dr. Sutherland for the Cranial Concept.

The primary and most significant difference between the practice of osteopathy in the cranial field and craniosacral therapy is the level of training of the practitioner. William Garner Sutherland, DO, introduced his cranial concept in 1929. Dr. Sutherland saw cranial osteopathy (OCMM, osteopathic cranial manual manipulation) as a modality of diagnosis and treatment to be provided by licensed physicians as part of a comprehensive treatment plan. As such, it is not merely a therapy, but an integral part of the physician's overall management of their patient's healthcare. Therapy is based on a protocol and not an individual diagnosis as opposed to a treatment, which is directed to a specific diagnosis for an individual. As osteopathic physicians specializing in neuromusculoskeletal medicine and providing osteopathic manual medicine, we are treating the patient's entire soma. We do not just treat a leg or just the head or just the shoulder. This integrative approach addresses the entire soma as one functional unit.

Craniosacral therapy (CST) is described as a "light touch therapy" that can be provided by a practitioner with as little as 8 days of training by the Upledger Institute or a weekend course somewhere else. The usual prerequisites for entrance into the CST program are having read Dr. Upledger's book and possession of any form of healthcare license, such as an audiologist, dietician, or massage therapist, although people without any healthcare license or training are sometimes also accepted. It is left to the states in which the craniosacral therapist resides to develop standards for its regulation.

Dr. Upledger was an osteopathic physician who took courses from Dr. Sutherland's students in cranial osteopathy in 1975, some 8 years before he established the Upledger Institute and published his first book on CST. Although Dr. Sutherland's concepts and techniques form the foundation of the CST model, it was Dr. Upledger's contention that it was he alone who pioneered and developed CST. Dr. Sutherland, on the other hand, credited his insights into the motion of the cranium to Andrew

Taylor Still, MD, the father of osteopathy. Dr. Still, for his part, took credit only for having discovered the science of osteopathy, saying "no human hand framed its laws." Authenticity and humility as a foundation within the profession of osteopathy, as exemplified by our teachers, acknowledges the credit our teachers deserve for their discoveries, insights, and teachings. Upledger teaching is also focused on technique as opposed to diagnosis, which leads the craniosacral therapist to treat the patient with a "one size fits all" approach as opposed to diagnosing and treating the somatic dysfunction uniquely present in each patient. Having said the above, there are some extremely talented craniosacral therapists who are of tremendous service and I have a great deal of respect for them. There is also gratitude for the Upledger Institute for creating a wide awareness of the cranium as a mobile structure. More people are now educated on the cranial concept and are thus seeking cranial care.

What are the benefits of osteopathic treatments during the ALF process?

Remember Gumby? He has no specific anatomical structure. He is pliable and bendable and when an injury occurs it creates a strain pattern in Gumby's body as he is bent and stretched in the specific pattern that expresses the physical form of the vector force of the injury.

The above image of Gumby represents a united structure moving as one functional unit. A compressive injury to the hip area can not only affect the hip motion but extend into the pelvis and leg to create movement dysfunctions and somatic tissue restrictions.

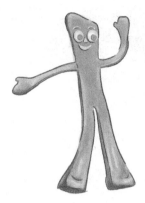

The older we get the more strain patterns we have to compensate for. Because of the decrease in elasticity and flexibility of the tissues with age, we also lose some of our adaptive capacities to move with these strain patterns. The longer a strain pattern is present the denser the tissue becomes within that pattern. As osteopaths our hands are trained to "read" the tissue textures and know the force, direction and timing of an injury. Our job is to remove the various tissue texture differences and create a more homogenous Gumby experience, so as to return him back to his original state of elasticity with an ease to bend. In the body as a river analogy, our job would be to remove the boulder in the river and allow the river to move freely without obstacles. In describing an osteopathic treatment to my new patients, I use the image of the body as a river with boulders inhibiting movement. Our hands are trained to hold the boulders in a way that transforms the rock back into sand that falls to the bottom of the river, thus allowing the fluids to move freely.

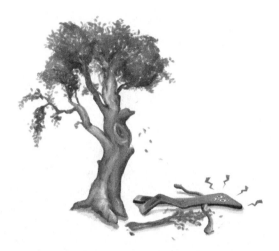

The vector force of an injury creates a pattern of somatic dysfunction according to the direction and magnitude of the compressive forces.

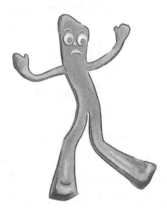

The above image is what Gumby might look like after an injury from a fall. The compressive forces impacted the soma. The areas of compressed and displaced tissue will create a pattern resembling the pattern of injury. These areas will have an increase in tissue density which is palpable. Osteopathic treatments address these areas of restriction and restore normal physiological tissue motion and function.

If Gumby falls from a height, like from a tree, the vector (the magnitude and direction) of the fall creates the shape and pattern of the compressive forces in the body. These compressive forces are "readable" or palpable by a well-trained osteopath. Gumby's "river" is going to express his unique compressive patterns created by the injuries his body has experienced. As injured tissue has less range of motion, his body will feel more dense and restricted to subtle or gross movement in those areas.

If Gumby grew with an anterior tongue thrust, now has an anterior open bite, can't eat a sandwich and needs an ALF appliance. In addition, he has fallen out of a tree with injuries to his neck, head and face. Gumby is going to need osteopathic treatment before he gets his ALF (in an ideal world!).

If one side of Gumby's neck, head and face has sustained an injury and the tissues are not pliable with a decrease in motion, the ALF appliance may not be able to unwind. As a consequence, the activation of the appliance will not create a symmetrical change in the tissues. As the ALF appliance is adjusted, the side or area of the face and cranium that has motion will expand to a greater degree and faster than the restricted side. Gumby will need osteopathic treatments to resolve his injuries before and during his ALF transformation.

ALF is an indirect osteopathic appliance (activates in the direction of ease) in the way that it simply augments motion that is present as well as stimulating growth and development. But depending on the extent of tissue restriction and hardening the ALF may not be able to unwind the tissue. Thus, it is essential for the patient to see an osteopathic physician to manually release the restricted area allowing the ALF to re-engage and create a symmetrical change. If the tissues are open and in a "Gumby state" then the ALF appliance will not create asymmetry when activated. This makes most adult ALF cases challenging cases that should consult with an osteopathic physician before ALF placement.

Osteopathic treatments pave a smooth path for the ALF process to be successful in a timely fashion with symmetrical growth. This piece of valuable information is often completely missed by many ALF dentists who have not had complete training in the ALF process.

It is ideal when the patient is able to receive osteopathic treatments along with the ALF adjustments. Not only for the optimal integrative experience but also to assure symmetrical growth. The treatments also significantly decrease treatment time needed to complete the ALF process, usually decreasing treatment time in half! In the end, this saves the patient's resources as dental appointments are usually more expensive than osteopathic appointments.

Many patients can do well with just the initial installation of the ALF appliance with regular adjustments. However, concomitant monthly osteopathic treatments as the ALF is adjusted would benefit patients with a birth history of any of the following: a prolonged labor, the use of Pitocin/epidural during birth, excessive molding of the head or bruising after birth, forceps or vacuum extraction, difficulty nursing, colicky, and/or spitting up. Also, if the patient has sustained any significant injuries/falls, headaches, back pain, developmental delays, recurrent ear or sinus infections, allergies, or asthma...just to name a few. These patients need to be treated by an osteopathic physician.

My website, www.drtashaturzo.com, has a list of cranial osteopathic physicians who have completed the ALF Educational Institute (AIE) residency program. At this time, most osteopathic physicians who have specialized in osteopathic manual medicine are not trained in the osteopathic-dental concept and have limited (to none) training in how to treat patients with the ALF appliances and communicate to ALF dentists. My hope is as this book educates the public, more practitioners will become trained in how to diagnose and treat craniofacial dysfunctions and treat with the ALF Approach (see Resources).

The ALF-trained orofacial myofunctional therapist

Many times the OMFT is the first ALF Approach team member a patient sees. Therefore, they are in the position to be able to identify the problems from a dental and neuromusculoskeletal perspective, educate the patient about the ALF Approach, and determine whether they need a referral to an ALF-trained cranial osteopath. Taking a complete birth and trauma history is essential for the ALF-trained OMFT, who can also assist with awareness of proper breathing and integrated reflexes. In this arena of looking at the whole being and working collaboratively, often the patient or parent feels reassured and relieved that there are solutions and that team members have the same understanding of the issues. While educating the patient, the OMFT starts the rapport needed to motivate and engage a patient in therapy. Patients often leave excited to get started and feel that they have been heard and now have a direction to resolve often overlooked etiologies that have worried or plagued them. They feel supported by team members that have gone beyond their standard education to find solutions to comprehensively treat their patients.

Customizing the treatment approach

Limitation of each profession in the ALF team

Each profession lacks important elements of a comprehensive treatment.

The DDS profession does not include:

- How postural changes create and are created by malocclusions
- How to assess and treat for cranial strain patterns and postural asymmetries
- How to assess for myofunctional dysfunction

- A complete history including birth, developmental and trauma to screen for difficult patients who need to be referred to an osteopath and OMFT
- Treating the underlying etiology of malocclusions
- The perspective of biotensegrity and thixotropy

The MFT profession does not include:

- Postural changes with myofunctional dysfunctions
- The taking of a complete history including birth, developmental and trauma to screen for difficult patients who need to be referred to an osteopath
- The perspective of biotensegrity and thixotropy

The DO profession does not include:

- How malocclusions are creating postural and cranial strain patterns
- How to assess for myofunctional dysfunction and when to refer to OMFT and an ALF DDS
- How to assess tongue function and tethered oral tissues and their effect on the cranium
- How to assess for airway dysfunctions
- How to treat the craniofacial cervical complex in relationship to oral function
- How to assess for temporomandibular dysfunction (TMD) in relationship to oral functions and the cranium
- How to treat TMD

The standard osteopathic educational curriculum does not include the interface of dentistry, orofacial myofunctional therapy and osteopathy and thus many of our patients receive limited assessments and treatment rather than a comprehensive integrative approach to craniofacial dysfunctions. The potency lies in collaborative courses where all three professions are learning and teaching with one another.

Should every patient with an ALF see both an orofacial myofunctional therapist and a cranial osteopathic physician?

In an ideal world, yes! But, as we all know, this is not reality, so below are some bullet points to help determine who should see who first. Once a patient is seeing an ALF-trained DDS, DO, or MFT, the hope is the team will communicate with one another guiding the patient through the transformational process.

Who should see a cranial osteopathic physician trained in the ALF Approach first?

- Any adult would be best served by starting with an osteopathic physician and treating the somatic dysfunctions present before applying the ALF appliance.

- Patients who have sustained significant physical trauma and/or have significant asymmetrical growth. For example, fractures, head injuries, back injuries, whiplash injuries, facial asymmetry or leg length discrepancy.

- Children who had a difficult birth or who have the following symptoms: colic, difficulty nursing, plagiocephaly, torticollis, difficulty gaining weight, fussy babies who have to be carried all the time, and excessive spitting up.

- Children with developmental delays, missed developmental milestones, or retained primary reflexes.

Who should see an ALF dentist first?

- If the palate is so narrow that the tongue cannot reach and rest in the palate, it is better to start sooner with an ALF appliance. If the patient is an adult or has had birth trauma/ injury, then osteopathy treatments will also be needed with OMFT to follow.

- If the patient's main issue is secondary to airway restriction that is creating acute health issues, then start with an ALF appliance right away with osteopathic treatments and OMFT to follow.

- If a patient has a crossbite, it is very important for the patient to seek ALF treatment. The crossbite will restrict the cranial bone motion and thus it is important for the osteopath to diagnose the crossbite on the first visit and then refer to an ALF DDS.

Who should see an orofacial myofunctional therapist first?

- Children with finger/thumb sucking habits. It's ideal to get the digits out of the mouth before starting the ALF process but not required.

- A skilled and well-trained OMFT can change the occlusions by integrating a functional swallow and neutral resting position of the tongue. In young children orofacial myofunctional therapy may solely be what is needed to redirect the malocclusion for better alignment.

CHAPTER 3

Cranial Birth Injuries, Facial Dysfunctions, and Malocclusions

What is considered a traumatic birth?

A traumatic birth should be considered if any of the following events occurred:

- Forceps or vacuum extraction

- Pitocin-assisted birth

- Shoulder dystocia (shoulders get stuck)

- C-section secondary to a failure to progress to a vaginal birth

- Excessive cranial molding/or bruising at birth

- More than two hours of pushing during the second stage of labor

- Difficulty breathing at birth/need for oxygen at birth

- Meconium present at birth

- Difficulty nursing after birth (could also be tongue-tied)

- Mother's milk supply is greater than baby's ability to swallow (baby difficulty organizing swallow)

- Difficulty nursing on both breasts with equal ease (points to torticollis and cervical somatic dysfunction)

- Infant lies with head always to one side (points to torticollis and cervical somatic dysfunction)

- Floppy musculoskeletal tone
- Colicky symptoms (see "Signs and symptoms of occipital condylar compression")
- Plagiocephaly (asymmetrical shaped newborn heads)
- Opisthotonos (rigidly arching backwards)
- Irritability
- Increased muscle tone or rigidity

Birth trauma and the connection to malocclusions

For most of us, birth is the most compressive experience our body encounters in a lifetime and these patterns of restrictive tissue can become the formative guiding vectors during growth and development. In an ideal world, which we all know is not what we live in, an osteopathic physician specializing in craniofacial dysfunction would treat every newborn until the rapid growing phase of life is complete. These birth tissue restrictions, somatic dysfunctions, occurring at the beginning of life, if they are not "released" the compression in the tissues can become not only a restrictive force to growth and development but also shapes and influences the directions of growth. The newborn cranium receives the greatest compressive forces as the uterine contractions drive the head into the opening cervix, forming the passageway to life. If there are obstacles to the opening of the cervix and pathway out of the mother's pelvis the baby's craniofacial cervical structure will mold and form to a shape in an attempt for survival which will accommodate the shape of the mother's passageway. Each person has had a unique experience of the specific compressive forces created by the relationship of mother's pelvis shape and accommodations to contractions with baby's position and capacity for cervix to open. C-section babies depending on the reason for the C-section can have a different compression story. If untreated these compressive vector forces can potentially influence growth and development. With osteopathic treatment and the ALF Approach these birth craniofacial cervical (and of course the rest of the body) compressive and restrictive forces can be released and normal growth and development can unfold into our greatest potential.

Human beings have large brains. That's the good news. The bad news is that the head is so big our mothers have to give birth to us before we are fully neurologically integrated to feed and move independently. Comparatively, we are born premature compared to other non-human primates. Other "non-human" mammals are born with the capacity to ambulate within minutes. Humans are born approximately one year before we are neurologically integrated enough to walk. Why is this? Because we have large brains and thus heads and we have to travel through our mother's pelvis before our heads are too big to fit. Thus we are born without the capacity to do anything except eat, sleep, poop and pee. It's an interesting compromise for intelligence!

The human body has adapted to this challenge by "floating" all the 37 craniofacial bones (including the ear bones and hyoid) within a membrane matrix, allowing the cranium to be moldable through fascia to the forces experienced during delivery. The bones of the infant's skull have not all ossified, and the bones are more numerous and more adaptive to the birth compressive forces. These bones are floating in membranous tissue, allowing maximum adaptive movement to conform to the mother's pelvis shape, capacity for her sacroiliac/pubic joints to widen, force and direction of mother's uterus contractions, and position of the baby in the pelvis.

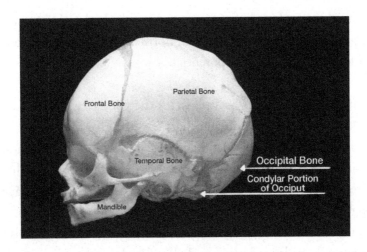

This is a photo of a newborn cranium. Notice the translucent fascia between the bones, which provide potential compressive space for the bones to move in order to accommodate birth compressive forces. (Photograph courtesy of Andrew Haltof, DO.)

For the baby presenting with head down occiput anterior (forward) posture (see image below) the area of most common and greatest compression is the occiput which can become compressed against the pubic symphysis or other non-yielding tissues. The joint between the occiput and the first cervical vertebra is often compromised because the occiput is commonly forced down into the cervical vertebra to compensate for the pressure through the cranium created by the mother's compressed, non-yielding soft tissue. If the baby's birth presentation is face-first and/ or a posterior presentation (also called "sunny-side up"), the face receives the most compressive forces. In a posterior presentation, the baby's face is descending with the bony pubic symphysis in front of the baby's face. The sacroiliac joints and sacrum have more capacity for expansion to create yielding soft tissue space for the passage of the baby's face with less compressive forces. The face is thus protected by facing towards the sacrum as the occiput descends against the bony pubic symphysis.

If the baby's face is compressed anteriorly (the front) there is a potential of creating midface compression during birth which could lead to midface and temporomandibular compression. These craniofacial compressions left untreated, have the potential to grow into maxillary deficiencies (crossbites) malocclusion and temporomandibular dysfunctions. The individual unique compressive forces during birth mold the baby's body which will compress to adapt to the space available as it strives to move to the outside world for its first breath and survival! Dentists and osteopaths trained in the craniofacial complex need to ask the birth stories to understand the complexities of the compressive forces that are shaping the patient's face and rest of the body. A difficult birth story will indicate a need for referral to the osteopathic physicians as soon as possible!

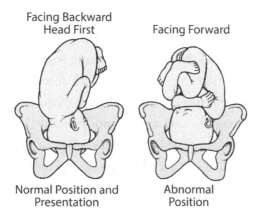

Facing Backward
Head First

Facing Forward

Normal Position and
Presentation

Abnormal
Position

The image on the left shows the baby facing towards the back of the pelvis. The capacity of the sacrum to rotate backwards and downwards increases the intra-pelvic dimension to accommodate space for the baby to traverse through. The yielding tissues of the sacroiliac joint (which connects the sacrum and pelvis) protect the face from excessive compression. The image on the right shows the baby's presentation with the face forward against the mother's pubic symphysis, increasing the potential for facial compression.

Let's talk details about the occipital bone, the "troublemaker" in birth injuries and how the occipital compressive birth forces are connected to facial growth dysfunction (malocclusions). At birth, the occipital bone exists as four separate bones surrounded by membranous tissues. The squamous portion of the occiput is the largest and forms most of the back of the head. There are two condylar portions of the occiput, on each side of which rest on top of the first cervical vertebrae, creating the occipitoatlantal (OA) joint. Just in front of the condylar portion of the occiput is the basilar portion, which forms a joint between the sphenoid and occipital bone called the sphenobasilar symphysis. A very important nerve runs between the basilar and condylar portion of the occiput called the hypoglossal nerve. This nerve is responsible for all the motor functions in the tongue.

The space between the two portions on the occiput (one on each side) is filled with fascia, and the bones are floating within a fascial matrix to optimize compensation to compressive birth forces. Three of the four pieces (the basilar and two condylar potions) of the occipital bone form a U-shape (see image below) and do not fuse until 8-9 years old! As the baby's head molds to the birth compressive forces, the area of least capacity for adaptation is at the OA joint. It's the first joint that the birth compressive forces encounter as the cranial bones are floating in fascia. Another way to put it is "the buck stops at the OA joint." Restrictions and compressions in this area create what osteopaths call occipital con-dylar compression syndrome. The symptoms are listed below and are the consequences of a compression or impingement to the cranial nerves 9-12 (glossopharyngeal, vagus, accessory, and hypoglossal nerves), which can occur at birth. These nerves all exit the cranium within fascia and next to the occipital bone within millimeters of one another, as the fol-lowing image shows.

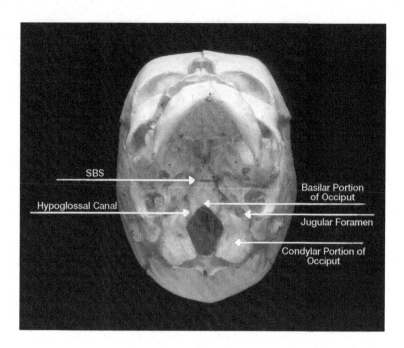

This is an image of a real fetal skull that clearly shows the four pieces of the occiput at birth. The hypoglossal canal is a space between the condylar portion of the occiput and the basilar portion of the occiput. These areas fuse together around the age of 8-9 years old. If there is an injury to the back of the head, either during birth or before the age of 8-9 years old, there can be a shear or displacement of these portions of occiput, creating a distorted hypoglossal canal and impingement of the hypoglossal nerve. Because this nerve innervates the muscle of the tongue, coordination of the swallowing process can be affected. Notice the jugular foramen is a space filled with fascia between the condylar portion of the occiput and the temporal bone. The cranial nerves 9-11 exit the cranium through this space between two cranial bones. These nerves are vulnerable to compression or impingement during the birth process as the bone shifts to accommodate compressive forces.

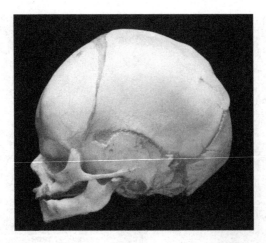

The above image is a fetal skull. Note the fascia (lighter translucent tissue) that connects the cranial bones and allows for molding of the cranium to occur during the birth process. This molding and reshaping of the cranium accommodates the compressive forces and protects the brain from injury.

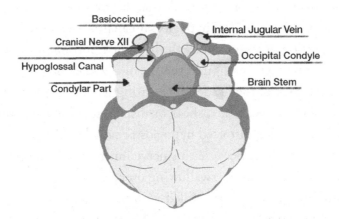

The above (inferior view) diagram of the occiput is drawn as if the patient is lying on the treatment table, with the practitioner's hands under the larger white area. The condylar parts are positioned forward in front of the practitioner's hands. The basiocciput is located in the middle of the cranium and articulates with the sphenoid bone. The white areas represent the four bones that make up the occiput. The squamous portion is the largest portion at the bottom of the picture. The two condylar parts and one basioccipital portion are labeled. The grey area represents the fascial tissues connecting the four parts of the occiput. Observe the hypoglossal nerve passing through the space between the condylar part and the basioccipital part of the occiput. This space becomes the hypoglossal canal when the occipital bones fuse into one bone around 8-9 years old. Also, note the position of the internal jugular vein which passes through the jugular foramen (not indicated in the image above), a space filled with fascia between the occipital and temporal bone. This foramen also houses cranial nerves 9-11, small arteries and the internal jugular vein. It is positioned just in front of the hypoglossal nerve and is also vulnerable to compression during the birth process.

Again the occipital condyle (the part of the bone in the back of your head that forms a joint with your first cervical vertebra) is formed by three separate bony parts of the occiput at birth with fascia filling the space between each of the bones. The space between two of these bones houses the most important nerve in facial growth and development, the hypoglossal nerve (cranial nerve 12). As the occipital bone is the most commonly injured cranial bone during a traumatic birth and the OA joint connecting the cranium with the first cervical vertebra is the area of least range of motion compared to the cranial bones floating in membrane we can conclude that this very small area becomes most vulnerable to distortions of membrane and displacement of bones. It is interesting to note that there is a membranous space between the occipital condylar portion of the occipital bone and the basiocciput portion of the occipital bone. Remembering that the occipital bone has not fused into one bone in the newborn but remains as four separate bones connected by membrane until 8-9 years old.[1] The space which connects the two is called the hypoglossal canal, which contains the hypoglossal nerve when the bones begin to fuse between eight and nine years old. Any distortion in the membranes or compression of the occipital bone during a traumatic birth, or an injury before 8-9 years old, can create a hypoglossal nerve impingement. As the bone fusion occurs after 9 years old, a distortion in the shape and size of the hypoglossal canal within the occipital bone can create an ongoing compression of the nerve and thus lack of coordination to the tongue.

What does this have to do with malocclusions? The hypoglossal nerve is the neural innervation for the control and movement of the tongue. If the tongue doesn't have the neuromuscular innervation to coordinate for its function, the tongue will default to a low lying position in the mouth as opposed to the facial growth and development favorable tongue to palate posture. Thus creating the experience of the palate not having the stimulation and molding from compression of the tongue for growth and development. The mid face will not develop forwards to its greatest potential. This is a predisposition for malocclusions and airway dysfunctions. Early signs of a tongue dysfunction are when an infant is unable to coordinate their tongue for nursing, lacks a strong sucking capacity, tires easily during nursing, or cannot accommodate the mother's milk supply. Many mothers think it's their fault that they produced too much milk and their baby couldn't swallow fast enough! This is usually not the case. The baby's swallowing capacity could be limited by the lack of optimal innervation by the hypoglossal nerve, creating the beginning of a dysfunctional swallowing pattern. This process will create facial growth and developmental dysfunctions (i.e. malocclusions).

Nursing is the earliest activity where we assess tongue function. All physicians treating in this area of medicine need to learn to diagnose early tongue function. All well-trained cranial osteopathic physicians (through the Cranial Academy[2]) know the signs and symptoms of condylar compression and are skilled in treating the area but many lack the knowledge of the connection between nursing dysfunctions and malocclusions and are limited in assessing tongue functions.

It is also important not to miss diagnosing a tongue-tie, which can present with similar symptoms as an impingement of the hypoglossal nerve. All cranial osteopathic physicians working with infants need to be trained to assess a tongue-tie (ankyloglossia). If there is a tight frenulum, the tissue needs to be released. It is best to work with a myofunctional therapist before and after the release to help strengthen the tongue muscle. Treatments with an osteopathic physician are important to release the areas of compensation for the tongue-tie. This becomes more imperative as the patient ages. Ankyloglossia is an area of rapidly changing new ideas. There are varying opinions and perspectives on the definition of a tongue-tie, or even what to call it, but learning to assess the function of the tongue helps guide us as to who needs a frenulum release as opposed to working with integrating and releasing restricted soft tissue compression from birth. We all have more to learn from each other as we (the practitioners) stay open and focus on collaborations.

Speech issues in children are another symptom associated with either a hypoglossal nerve impingement or ankyloglossia, or both. A referral to a cranial osteopath and myofunctional therapist is imperative which usually clears up the speech issues. Rarely, but sometimes, a referral to a speech therapist is needed.

Signs and symptoms of occipital condylar compression

- Difficulty sucking
- Difficulty swallowing
- Frequent spitting up
- Reflux
- Respiratory problem
- Torticollis (wry neck). Early signs are difficulty nursing on one side indicating there is a cervical restriction.
- Arching of the back (opisthotonus)
- Colic

- Constipation
- Bloating
- Flatulence
- Insomnia
- Irritability

If the infant shows any of the above symptoms, they should see a cranial osteopathic physician to assess and treat the cranium. If you have had a history of any of the above as an infant, it is never too late to be treated. An adult patient who had the above symptoms as an infant and/or a history of a traumatic birth is considered a complicated ALF patient and needs to see a cranial osteopathic physician first before the placement of the ALF appliances.

Occipital condylar compression and the colicky baby

The typical presentation of a baby with occipital condylar compression created by increased compressive forces on the occiput at birth is a "colicky" or fussy baby with gas, reflux, spitting up, difficulty self-soothing, sleeping and sometimes difficulty nursing. Any or just one of these symptoms could be present. These are the babies that need to be treated by cranial osteopathy immediately. Let's go through the neurophysiology of the above symptoms and explain how these symptoms are associated with birth injury and malocclusions.

There is another very important space that lies between the temporal and occipital cranial bones. It's called the jugular foramen and it is where some very important structures pass through. This foramen is a space between the occiput and the temporal bones of the cranium. The space is represented in the above diagram by the blue region. The glossopharyngeal nerve, vagus nerve, and accessory nerve are the cranial nerves that pass through this space between the two cranial bones, the occiput and the temporal bone (see images above.) Two venous structures and the glymphatics system responsible for draining the central nervous system along with two small arteries also pass through the jugular foramen. As the cranial bones shift to accommodate the birth compressive forces, the volume of the space between these two bones can change, creating a potential fascial strain with compression to the vital structures that pass through. Nerves are very sensitive to compression and even with a small fascial strain in the tissues around a nerve, they will be activated in a dys-synchronization pattern, leading to a dysfunction at the end point of the neural innervation.

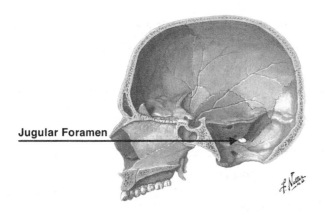

Jugular Foramen

The glossopharyngeal nerve activates some of the swallowing muscles and is the sensory innervation to the back of the tongue for taste, upper pharynx, and the temporomandibular joint. The nerve also has other functions. A compression and dysregulation of this nerve can create a dysfunction in swallowing. The vagus nerve (10th cranial nerve) is the longest nerve in the body and is called the "king of the nerves" because of its vast effects in the body. Sections in Chapter 6 present more detail. This nerve is largely responsible for the action of swallowing as well as gut and brain functions. The spinal accessory nerve (11th cranial nerve) is responsible for the contraction of the sternocleidomastoid and trapezius muscles. These muscles play a large role in flexing and extending the head, bending the head to the same side, and rotating the head to the opposite side. When these muscles are over-contracted, the condition is called torticollis and/or "wry neck."

What is the potential consequence of compression of these cranial nerves? Basically, it can present as a colicky baby with symptoms of irritability, bloating and gas, constipation, difficulty nursing and swallowing, as well as torticollis. It is also worth noting here that facial growth and development will be impacted by the dysregulation of the cranial nerves 9-11, as the swallowing patterns will be less than optimal, resulting in atypical swallowing patterns.

The symptoms of jugular foramen syndrome or Vernet's syndrome are the same as the symptoms of occipital condylar compression but to a lesser degree of severity. Vernet's syndrome is characterized by paresis (paralysis) of the glossopharyngeal, vagal, and accessory nerve with or without the hypoglossal nerve.[3] [4] [5]

Symptoms of this syndrome are consequences of this paresis. As such, in an affected patient, you may find:

- Dysphonia/hoarseness
- Soft palate dropping
- Deviation of the uvula towards the normal side
- Dysphagia
- Loss of sensory function from the posterior 1/3 of the tongue (cranial nerve 9)
- Decrease in the parotid gland secretion (cranial nerve 9)
- Loss of gag reflex
- Sternocleidomastoid and trapezius muscles paresis (cranial nerve 11)

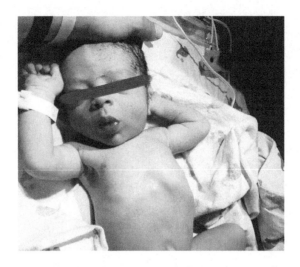

Above is a newborn with torticollis and history of a difficult birth of four hours of pushing. Also note the plagiocephaly (misshapen head) in the below photo as a consequence of the compressive forces of birth. Note in the above photo the asymmetry of the mandible. The right mandible is sloped with a straight line down to the left. The neck is rotated to the right. The below picture expresses the comfortable position of his hand on the right mandible, which most likely is the position he grew in utero. The baby most likely grew with his hand on this right face, which directed the growth of his mandible. He also most likely descended into the pelvis with his hand in this position as a consequence of the difficult labor.

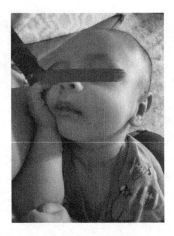

This child has been treated since birth with osteopathy and the cranium is mostly symmetrical but the mandible still deviates to the left when opening. The early intervention will help to redirect the growth patterns of the cranium and face. However, as the face grows out from under the cranium it may still have an asymmetric presentation. He most likely will need the ALF Approach as early as 3 years old to redirect the growth of the mandible and occlusion.

CHAPTER 4

Orofacial Myofunctional Disorders

by Kathy Winslow, BS, RDH, COM™

What are orofacial myofunctional disorders?

Orofacial myofunctional disorders (OMDs) include any or a combination of the following:

- Lack of lip seal

- Mouth breathing

- Low tongue rest position

- Parafunctional habits (thumb, finger, object sucking, nail biting, lip licking and biting, clenching, and bruxism)

- Increased and decreased vertical dimensions of facial development

- Chewing disorders, messy eating, open mouth chewing, food/ texture aversions

- Atypical swallowing (tongue thrusting), aerophagia, drooling

- Restricted labial or lingual and buccal frenums (tethered oral tissues)

- Swollen nasal passages, adenoids, and large tonsils from oral breathing, allergies, and or laryngopharyngeal acid reflux (LPRD) may also contribute to the maladaptive dysfunctions such as tongue thrusting and mouth breathing

- Jaw thrusting during speech

- High incidence of speech problems.[1] The /s/ sound is the most common, others are /z/, /sh/, /ch/, /l/, /t/, /n/, /d/ and /r/.

111

What is the prevalence and impact of OMDs?

Although numerous studies have evaluated the prevalence of tongue thrusting, there are very few surveillance studies on the prevalence and impact of OMDs. One paper stated "The frequency of myofunctional disorders was statistically significantly higher in children with increased maxillary overjet, frontal open bite, lateral crossbite and mandibular prognathism, and there was a statistically significant increase in the prevalence of orofacial dysfunctions and oral habits from primary to mixed dentitions."[2]

From what I see in practice, the prevalence is higher than has been reported and there is a need for more formal research in this area. With sleep apnea and sleep disordered breathing on the rise, often correlating with neurocognitive issues like ADHD, Alzheimer's, and Parkinson's,[3-7] further investigation of causation is necessary. Poor craniofacial development is often a common thread with airway issues and orofacial myofunctional therapy may be an integral part of prevention, treatment, and stabilization for desired outcomes.[8-14] The most important part of an OMD assessment is to identify the causes and obstacles that initiate and contribute to having an OMD. Multiple aspects of a patient's health history, including *in utero* experience, delivery, trauma, diet, habits, environment, inflammation, posture, and even dentistry performed, must be evaluated.

We have evolved and are naturally programmed to have adequate jaw space for 32 teeth, a beautifully balanced face (normal craniofacial shape and jaw relationships) that allows for normal function, proper growth and development with a structurally sufficient patent airway. Unfortunately, there are a plethora of etiologies that often make these functionally healthy and beautiful outcomes elusive. Daniel Lieberman postulates that the human skull is changing faster than the normal rate of evolution would dictate.[15]

As stated in Enlow's Essentials of Facial Growth: "The genetic and functional *determinants* of a bone's development (i.e. the origin of growth-regulating signals) reside in the composite of soft tissues, that turn on or turn off, or speed up or slow down, the histogenic actions of the osteogenic connective tissues. Growth is not *"programmed"* within the bone itself or enclosing membranes. The *"blueprint"* for the design, construction, and growth of a bone thus lies in the *muscles, tongue, lips, cheeks, integument, mucosae, connective tissues, nerves, blood vessels, airway, pharynx, the brain as an organ mass, tonsils, adenoids, and so forth,* all of which provide information signals that pace the histogenic tissues producing a bone's development."[16]

It has been well documented by Van Der Klaauw[17] and Moss[18] [19] that the stomatognathic system is influenced by the constant interactions between the functional motion of soft tissues and the effects on the developing skeletal structures. Form and function are reciprocal and hence the importance of identifying OMDs and their etiologies as early as possible is paramount. The craniofacial complex develops rapidly, therefore catching problems early and removing the obstacles for proper growth and development often requires a team approach.

Explained by the authors of the text *Contemporary Orthodontics,* due to the "rapid growth exhibited by children during the primary dentition years it would seem that treatment of jaw discrepancies by growth modification should be successful at a very early age. If treated from ages 4-6 when rapid growth occurs, significant improvements in skeletal discrepancies can be accomplished in a short period of time." Treatment can still be beneficial and required for older patients as well. Dr. Kevin Boyd, a pediatric dentist, has devoted his time and practice to researching anthropology for what craniofacial norms were before environmental influences have shaped the functional and structural outcomes we see today. Many airway-focused dentists are pioneering new ways to augment derailed normal development to provide better structural and functional health.

In the 1980s, Darick Nordstrom, DDS, took the principles of the Crozat appliance to develop the ALF appliance. Dr. Nordstrom relied on osteopathic feedback to refine the ALF appliance to create a biocompatible dental appliance. In 1996, Drs. Nordstrom and Turzo began collaborating on the ALF design to optimize function for each patient individually. Dr. Turzo met James Bronson, DDS, in 2012 at a conference at which she and Dr. Nordstrom were teaching and invited him to treat ALF patients in her office in Santa Cruz, CA. Dr. Bronson also saw the potential in delivering this transformative, supportive, and versatile osteopathic appliance to young children and adults, as well as the need to train more professionals.

Dr. Bronson, Dr. Turzo, and I have been fortunate enough to teach together how the team approach is essential to treat and finish cases. We rely on each other's focus of expertise to customize treatment for our patients. The functional dentist uses the appliance to unwind cranial strain patterns and gently redirect the growth with orthotropic enhancement and correction of malocclusion. Osteopathy is essential for enabling the body to adapt to change and to be medically receptive. The orofacial myofunctional therapist is responsible for transforming behavioral habits and functional incongruencies, and integrating them into new corrected postural and functional patterns that enhance proper growth and provide stability. It appears that the ALF neuro-reflexively mimics the tongue to the brain stem and provides the biomechanical stimulation for bone growth. The tongue both reflexes up to the appliance and activates it with every correct swallow. The swallow and postures still often need to be rehabilitated with myofunctional therapy to correct the dysfunctions. The ALF provides an unwinding with its tensegrity, support, and flexibility assisting to decompress the midline sutures. Having the tongue up in the palate also accomplishes this. The whole tongue postured in the palate will affect all three postural mechanisms. Our anatomy needs symmetry to organize the anti-gravity mechanisms. Our jaw correlates with the vestibular systems left and right. Eighty percent of our movements are actively creating asymmetry and are strongly dependent on head, tongue, and temporomandibular joint (TMJ) position. The tongue is the regulator of all of these things. The ALF also helps the whole body function in more stable 3-dimensional events.

The fact that the ALF does not interfere with tongue space is a plus; the gentle approach is even better for all ages, especially the little ones. Allowing for tongue space is one of the most attractive elements of the ALF appliance from a myofunctional standpoint because it can be used in conjunction with treatment, allowing for the proprioception created between the tongue and the palate. It is important that the ALF is used properly initially as an osteopathic appliance rather than an orthodontic appliance. Identifying the professionals such as an osteopathic physician who may intervene at critical times by sequencing the assistance needed requires an understanding and identification of the etiologies and compensations that occur in response. Etiologies such as altered (in-utero influences, birth/delivery), lack of or compensatory breastfeeding, absence of nasal breathing, tethered oral tissues, retained reflexes, poor chewing, swallowing, and rest postures, as well as habits and trauma, may all contribute to poor craniofacial development, malocclusion, SDB (sleep disordered breathing) and even poor posture. These professionals must be aware of what treatments apply, when, and with whom. A myriad of comorbidities such as SDB, sleep apnea, ADHD, neurocognitive and behavioral morbidity in children with sleep disorders may result if oral dysfunction is not treated early, which can be serious and may be avoided or abated when attended to.[20] [21]

The perfect team consists of an orofacial myofunctional therapist treating the OMDs, an osteopath providing cranial and whole-body treatment with medical supervision, and a functional dentist/ orthodontist utilizing the ALF, where one, two, or all three practitioners may be required to change the course dysmorphology. Other professionals may be required as well, such as ENTs, allergists, oral surgeons, periodontists, physical therapists, and occupational therapists.

Orofacial myofunctional therapy (OMFT) focuses on tongue rest and functional patterns with a lip seal and habit elimination. A good part of an OMFT program may involve coordinating and toning the musculature for rest, eating, drinking and even functional speech patterning. Also in the scope of the OMFT is assisting with the correction of oral phase dysphagia (problems with using the mouth, lips and tongue to control food or liquid). Speech disorders such as articulation errors, apraxia, aphasia, dysarthria and any pharyngeal dysphagia swallowing disorders are treated by trained speech pathologists. Along with the foundational components of myofunctional therapy there may be many other factors such as restricted frenulum that often need to be addressed.[22]

When addressing myofunctional treatment approaches regarding a restricted frenum, I often ask the question: Why bother revising a restricted frenulum without changing the function and postures to allow for the full benefit of the procedure? Is there enough room for the tongue to fit, in order to help maintain the optimal elevation of the whole tongue into the palate once the restriction is elevated and rehabilitated? Protocols of coordinating and strengthening the muscles, starting functional corrections, initiating nasal breathing, as well as promoting thinning of tissue with musculature and blood vessels retreating, are goals that allow the professional providing the revision easier access to the tissues to be treated with a release. It is also paramount to make sure midline and cranial nerves are integrated. Fascial release mediated by an osteopath is ideal as well, especially in the cervical, hyoid, and diaphragm areas.

The postoperative exercises are reviewed prior to the frenectomy so that the brain is familiar with the neuromuscular pathways to do the postoperative exercises, despite the existing restrictions. I follow the patients post operatively and every 2-4 days for several weeks during the healing phase to support them. Osteopathic treatments should be done both before and after the frenectomy as well if at all possible. As my colleague Patricia Pine, RDH, COM™ stated in her book *Please Release Me*, the orofacial myofunctional therapist is the quarterback in the multidisciplinary team. Great results are achieved by selecting the correct specialist and procedure, with concurrent supervised and supported pre-/post-op exercises, and completing the rehabilitation of the function and rest posture.

"Positive behavior modification and motivational therapy are used to eliminate harmful oral habits such as prolonged pacifier, thumb or finger sucking; fingernail, cheek, or lip biting; tongue sucking; and clenching/grinding of the teeth."[23] It is often necessary to both identify and eliminate the etiology that may have been the source of the habit that is originally a compensation to create stability. The underlying goal the habits may be providing could be to open the airway, enlist the parasympathetic and limbic system by using the thumb or fingers to seal the oral complex and establish nasal breathing. Sometimes there may be an inability to elevate the tongue.

Endorphins are produced when the nasal palatine area is stimulated (the spot) during normal tongue function. The digit is substituted to replace the stimulation the tongue would have been providing in optimal function. Nocturnal bruxism is often a parafunctional habit to maintain the airway during sleep. Oral breathing creates a negative relationship between the pharynx and upper esophageal sphincter. Upper airway resistance syndrome (UARS) and sleep apnea can create desensitization of the sensory awareness as well as reduction in tone because of persistent negative airway pressure on the musculature. Oropharyngeal exercises that target the tongue, soft palate, lateral pharyngeal wall and lips were used in the Guimaraes and colleagues 2009 study.[24] The study concluded that there was reduced pharyngeal collapsibility, resulting in improved daytime sleepiness symptoms, smaller neck circumference, reduction in snoring, and apnea hypopnea index (AHI) scores.

Upper airway muscles have increased activity when solely nasal breathing is present.[25]

Nasal breathing also provides nitric oxide made in the nasal sinuses responsible for cleansing the air and improving endothelium elasticity and function. Orofacial myofunctional therapy may provide additional assistance in improving sleep/breathing results.[26] [27]

History of orofacial myofunctional disorders

Edward Angle, the father of modern orthodontics, stated in 1907: "We are just beginning to realize how common and varied are vicious habits of the lips and tongue, how powerful and persistent they are in causing and maintaining malocclusion, how difficult they are to overcome and how hopeless is success in treatment unless they are overcome."[28]

Between 1918 and 1950, a series of therapeutic exercises were developed to correct and improve these disorders. In 1960 Walter Straub had a theory that bottle feeding caused the "perverted" swallow. He developed a series of exercises to correct the swallow. He lectured based on 500 case records.

OMFT had struggled in the 1980s to be identified as mainstream, striving for more research to verify its significance and importance as a potential modality (in striving) for proper development and health. The latest international research from the Sleep Medicine Division of Stanford University, as well as the Department of Otorhinolaryngology, Ophthalmology and Head and Neck Surgery of the University of Sao Paulo, and Dr. Kevin Boyd, to name a few, are finding new relationships and evidence worth noting.

OMFT is now a hot topic of research to aid not only craniofacial development and airway issues that may relate to sleep apnea as well as the sequelae and comorbidities that are associated with the structural and functional issues inherent with OMDs.[29]

In the 1970s, the late Dr. Christian Guilleminault identified sleep disorders even in children and has been a pioneer in the medical and dental field for research to aid professionals in finding solutions for these all-too-prevalent comorbidities that are caused by sleep-disordered breathing. He identified OMFT as one of the modalities to assist in correcting these problems.[30]

A meta-analysis and systematic review of literature published (done) by M. Camacho, MD, et al, concluded that "Current literature demonstrates that myofunctional therapy (OMFT) decreases the apnea-hypopnea index in 50% of the adults (9 studies) and 62% of the children (2 studies). Lowest O2 saturation, snoring, and sleepiness outcomes improved in adults. Following tonsil and adenoidectomy in children with (OMFT) they had no recurrent OSA 5 years later as compared to those without (OMFT). Myofunctional therapy could serve as an adjunct to other obstructive sleep apnea treatments."[31]

Current causes of OMDs

The unintended consequences of convenience in today's world have contributed to OMDs. Narrower pelvises, shared space (twins), and a fetal head engaged low in the birth canal too early, are just some of the conditions that may prevent normal fetal movements that aid training the tongue reflexively with normal activity in the womb and may contribute to poor tongue function postpartum. Normal flexion, extension and rotational work that the fetus must do to get through the canal, along with the paced contractions and the squeeze and initiation of the first breath, set the stage for proper reflexes and functional development for breathing. Birthing practices such as the use of Pitocin, epidurals, and C-sections may be necessary but alter the normal process may pose problems such as retained reflexes.

The "birth crawl," which is the skin-to-skin contact with the newborn crawling up the mother's belly and latching onto the breast, is required to aid in the head and neck movements and reflexes. When a suboptimal labor and delivery occurs, the nervous system may be locked into fight or flight (Moro reflex and or tendon guard) and often the baby is swaddled and handed to the mother without being able to work through those reflexes. Inappropriately active reflexes and aberrant tonal patterning may deny one from progressing onto the next functioning level, and must be addressed by professionals with extra training with either cranial nerve integration and/or reflexes. Six of the twelve cranial nerves are involved in sucking. Excessive or prolonged compression on the cranium, or the absence of it in the case of C-sections, may impact the cranial nerves' ability to perform optimally. In my opinion, in an ideal world an osteopath would be present in every labor and delivery room to help mitigate and unwind these strain patterns exerted on the cranium during delivery. This could help to integrate the reflexes that may be inhibiting the baby's progression in the hierarchy of functional levels.[32]

These unevolved reflexes may hinder OMFT outcomes if not addressed initially. Mis-mapping, or our brain's inability to take the sensory input and deliver it to the appropriate body part for function and sensation, is found with cranial nerve dysfunction and must also be addressed. As in Hebb's Axiom: What fires together wires together. The good news is that our brains also learn from movement. The brain needs to feel safe in order to learn.

Maxine Haller, OT/L, suggests a sequence of stimulatory nerve patterns:

1. Input of passive movement (movement done by the provider)

2. Progression from passive to active (ability to repeat movements – from the *brainstem to the cerebellum*)

3. More sophisticated active movements (repeat and control the actions – from the *cerebellum to the basal ganglia*)

4. Judgement or choice of when (timed)

Basic function needs to be a choice. It is essential to access the building blocks that reflexes provide for synergistic coordinated movements.

By targeting the areas that need stimulation with movements of flexion, extension, and rotation we can turn on the wiring and reset it. The development of movement is an evolution according to Brunnstom's stroke rehab approach. Similarly myofunctional therapy aims to provide awareness, placement, stability, endurance, and muscle memory, with a corrected functional pattern retained. I feel that OMFT, with its neuromuscular exercise training, inherently provides and creates neuroplasticity by changing the brain with movement and repatterning in order to change the function.

Sucking is one of our deepest and most primal reflexes; if a baby isn't sucking at birth, the brain doesn't know how to keep the throat safe. Only stimulation between the hard and soft palate trains the neck and brain to learn the first and second phases of sucking deeply. The second phase of involuntary control and regulation informs the brain about the ability to protect the throat for swallowing, according to Svetlana Masgutova, founder of the Masgutova Neurosensorimotor Reflex Integration (MNRI).

Proper nursing (not compensatory) influences optimal growth and development of the craniofacial respiratory complex as noted by Jennifer Tow, a holistic IBCLC. Absence or early cessation of breastfeeding may prevent the tongue's proper function and rest posture that develop the midface, maxilla, premaxilla, and nasal airway. The sucking action translates the mandible forward and back to help develop the lower jaw.

The posterior suction from a tongue that can move and function normally has the pressure and suction on the area near the sphenobasilar symphysis. This helps develop the floor of the cranium so that the rest of the face and airway is suspended.

As Mao, Wang, and Kopher observed, "...mechanical forces regulate sutural growth by inducing sutural mechanical strain...oscillatory strain likely turns on genes and transcription factors that activate cellular machinery via mechanotransduction pathways."[33]

The trend in infant feeding has changed how our jaws have developed in the last 350 years with industrialization, mechanization and agriculture. Breast-feeding and baby-led weaning encourage optimal jaw and facial development conducive to healthy breathing. "Our nutritionally deficient and soft diets are not providing the nourishment for stronger bone development."[34]

Chewing nutritious unprocessed food develops the jaws (the muscle action on the developing bone).[35] [36] Children's oral volume is "tight packed" until the teeth come in and "food for fun until age one" is a motto to remember.[37]

Nutritious breast milk is usually sufficient until age one. However, the child needs to practice the sensory motor movements of gnawing and chewing not only to aid in growth and development but to practice, so that when the teeth erupt creating more oral volume space they won't choke. These functions help prevent malocclusion and provide a structurally adequate nasal floor and pharyngeal space to breathe, free of inflamed tonsils and adenoids, and good alignment of the spine. Our diets and environmental influences may contribute to allergies, and inability to nasal breathe. Swollen turbinates, deviated septums (usually caused by poor craniofacial development), polyps, inflammation that may be caused by silent reflux into the upper oral pharynx and nasal complex may force oral breathing with poor craniofacial outcomes.[38]

In a three-dimensional study, the influence of snoring, mouth breathing and apnea on facial morphology in late childhood concluded that retrusive jaws, narrow and retruded maxillas, a less prominent narrow nose, and steep mandibular angles with longer facial dimensions are diagnostic features of sleep disordered breathing (SDB) that may require referrals to other specialists for clinical symptoms related to SDB as well.[39]

Resolving the etiologies contributing to the dysfunction so that lip seal and continuous nasal breathing are the norm is one of the primary goals and may require numerous specialists to achieve.[40]

Epigenetic influences prompting changes in our physiology such as DNA methylation may be contributing to changes in our anatomy such as restricted labial and lingual frenulums.[41] These in turn restrict function and may also contribute to insufficient craniofacial development and malocclusions.[42]

There is an increased prevalence of tongue-ties, probably because of increased awareness (more mothers are trying to breastfeed), hereditary contributions, and the epigenetic influences of environment (chemicals, flame retardant, glyphosate toxins) and diet.[43]

Common causes of OMDs

There can be many factors that can cause an orofacial myofunctional disorder, including:

- Improper oral habits such as thumb or finger sucking, cheek/nail biting, tooth clenching/grinding
- Restricted nasal airway due to enlarged tonsils/adenoids and/or allergies, and facial trauma to the nose
- Structural or physiological abnormalities such as short lingual frenum (tongue attachment to the floor of the mouth)

- Neurological or developmental abnormalities
- Hereditary predisposition to some of the above factors
- Trauma, birth, and other injuries

What are some potential consequences of OMDs?

Abnormal functional activities, habit patterns, and poor oral postures may create an environment that can disrupt dental eruption patterns in children. Sub-optimal jaw growth/position, and malocclusion may lead to an abnormal facial profile. This poor craniofacial development may cause other problems with the airway and temporomandibular joint.

The orofacial myofunctional therapist may aid in correcting the behavioral and muscular dysfunction contributing to temporomandibular dysfunction (TMD). In 2005, Castelo noted in his findings that only atypical swallowing was positively related to TMD and that oral non-nutritive habits were not directly related to TMD.[44] However, digit sucking promotes atypical swallowing. I do believe that the oral habits during development may also hinder the proper development of the TMJ complex, due to the altered oral postures during habit activity. The incorrect function is an adaptation that further promotes the dysfunction. TMD treatment must always be in collaboration with the dentist, osteopath, and other appropriate professionals.[45]

Forward head posture (often as a result of poor craniofacial development, and trying to open the airway) is often associated with TMD and neck issues. Osteopathy and/or physical therapy may be necessary.[46]

Chronic open mouth rest posture may create increased vertical height of the face, recessive chin, and hypotonic or flaccid lips. This downward, backward growth (rather than downward and forward) may contribute to airway obstructions and sleep-disordered breathing, upper airway restrictive syndrome (UARS), and sleep apnea.[47]

The anterior face changes but so does the suspended pharyngeal airway. A deviated septum, sinusitis, and a high narrow palate that have invaded the nasal space can create a negative pressure that may cause reflux to add to the inflammation. Behavioral problems and academic and social challenges often are associated with sleep disordered breathing (SDB).[48]

Concerning non-cardiovascular morbidities: neurocognitive impacts with neurobehavioral consequences show that 30% of all children with frequent and loud snoring manifest significant inattention and hyperactivity. Cognitive deficits in learning, mental processing, and executive functioning in children occur with obstructive sleep apnea syndrome (OSAS). These may be persistent in adolescence and adulthood even after resolution of snoring if the initial OSAS is untreated.[49] [50]

Nocturnal enuresis is another co-morbidity associated with obstructive sleep apnea (OSA) with recent results showing that decreased in frequency of events or complete cessation of enuresis after OSA has been successfully treated.

These are just some of the examples of the many different outcomes of poor oral postures and functions. OMDs often play a role in open mouth chewing, drooling, digit habits, speech issues, and mouth breathing, all of which may lead to social embarrassment, as well as significant health issues.

What is orofacial myofunctional therapy?

Orofacial myofunctional therapy (OMFT) involves an individualized regimen of therapeutic passive and resistive oral and facial muscle exercises. It focuses on the neuromuscular re-education of the orofacial complex to normalize and correct chewing and swallowing patterns as well as tongue, jaw, and lip resting postures. Abnormal rest postures may contribute to malocclusion and improper craniofacial development and may also play a role in the development of airway issues."[51]

Why orofacial myofunctional therapy works!

Case 1 – Habit elimination digit program with myofunctional therapy.

Initial
6 years
old

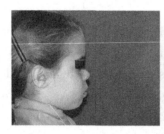

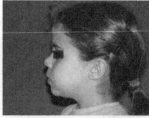

30 days
no thumb

- Thumbsucking with habit elimination: Faces have a chance to develop properly

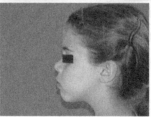

2 months

Initial   30 Days   2 months

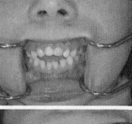 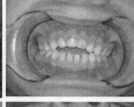 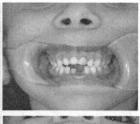

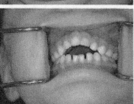 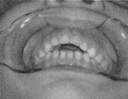 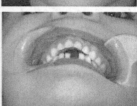

Case 2 – Mouth breathing, low postured tongue, and anterior tongue thrust. Breathing restoration and myofunctional therapy.

Progress in facial tone and symmetry

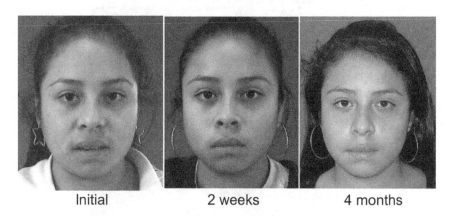

Initial   2 weeks   4 months

Initial Ventral view
Anterior Tongue Thrust

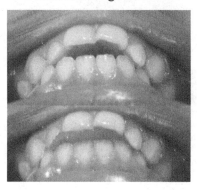

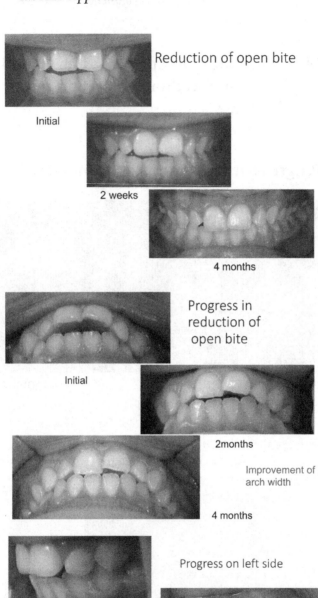

Reduction of open bite

Initial

2 weeks

4 months

Progress in
reduction of
open bite

Initial

2months

Improvement of
arch width

4 months

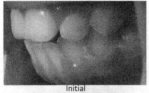

Progress on left side

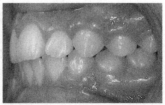

Initial

4 months

The tongue posturing low in the mouth interposed between or on top of the mandibular arch during rest and thrusting forward (pictured above) impedes the eruption of the teeth and alters the bony structure. This may create either a Class II or, if sitting in the lower arch, possibly a Class III occlusion. The tongue thrusting jams the jaw back and the facial nerves and muscles are used to stabilize the jaw to keep the food or saliva in the oral cavity during the swallow instead of the muscles of mastication and proper use of the tongue as well. The tongue thrusting may also be bilateral, unilateral, or inside of the mouth into the teeth, that may contribute to malocclusion, TMD, and cervical issues.

OMFT provides an integrated, compassionate approach to educating and motivating clients to achieve orofacial muscle balance and proper function.

Muscles respond better to regular and consistent exercise. OMFT is a non-invasive therapy that helps train the muscles of the face and tongue through simple exercises taught by a specialist who can customize the individual's therapy. Teamwork and motivation is paramount.

OMFT is an exercise program that is fun and takes only three to five minutes (some instances longer) two to three times a day. 30-minute resting postures may also be employed. Eating correctly takes longer but eating is for most of us a daily routine.

Therapy takes approximately 10 to 17 visits and sometimes more, over a 6- to 12-month interval.

Goals of orofacial myofunctional therapy

Palatal tongue rest posture, lip seal, nasal breathing, and a corrected chewing and swallow are the fundamental goals of OMFT. Relaxation of the muscles of expression and elimination of facial grimaces during deglutition are also required. Parafunctional habits are transferred to constructive habits or eliminated. Proper head and body alignment is a goal and may require other practitioners as well. With additional training in restorative breathing and retained reflexes (that may be inhibiting the progression of corrected function and rest postures), identification, restoration, and integration of normal breathing and age aligned appropriate response of reflexes can be done prior or concurrently. When impediments to proper breathing and function are present, referrals may be necessary.

Another primary goal of OMFT should be to establish or recapture a normal freeway space open at rest. A normal range of 2-3 mm at the molars is desired. When making a referral to an OMFT for post-orthodontic relapse, a clinician should evaluate three rest postures: the freeway space (the normal interocclusal rest position is 2-3 mm between the molars and 3-5 mm between the incisors), the rest posture of the tongue (either up or down, but not interdental), and whether there is lip competence (lips together/seal without strain).

The overall goal of OMFT is to correct maladapted postural and functional archetypes, thus integrating and habituating the new normal pattern. "This re-education process is gradual and must be assimilated over a period of time long enough for it to become the more efficient and dominantly established pattern. OMFT works as an adjunct to dental care, aiding the dentist and orthodontist in achieving and maintaining the optimal functional aspects of treatment,"[52] as well as helping stabilize osteopathic treatment by removing the aberrant muscle functions that may be contesting the homeostasis that the treatment provided.

At completion of therapy, it is so much fun to observe the perplexed look on their faces when asked to swallow incorrectly and it is evident they can't remember how to or even manage to swallow improperly. Correcting OMD helps provide long-term homeostasis for more successful orthodontic outcomes, and aids muscular TMD and other oral health therapies as well. Bringing harmony to the orofacial muscles provides a stable environment for proper growth, development, and function.

I also feel the role of the OMFT is to be the educator of OMDs and resulting symptoms, and a collaborator connecting the patients to the professionals that can help them.

This profession can be extremely gratifying when you've helped the patient, and often whole families achieve better health. My motto is the 3 R's: Recognize, Respond, and Refer. Only then can you identify, prevent, facilitate, and stabilize treatment. "Stability of these results is dependent on the elimination of the OMDs to establish harmonious muscle function" according to the authors Proffit, et al.[53]

Global goals for the orofacial myofunctional therapist are to educate, identify, prevent, facilitate, stabilize, and collaborate.

Qualified OMFT practitioners

Licensure as a health professional such as a dental hygienist, speech-language pathologist, dentist, or physician is required for any post-graduate training in orofacial myofunctional therapy (OMFT). Physical therapists have knowledge of the cranial cervical complex and also may work with the TMJ. Some have acquired training in OMFT. I have found that my experience as a dental hygienist was an excellent foundation for this specialty.

There is additional training in breathing restoration that many orofacial myofunctional therapists have done to aid in changing the physiology and behavior that may contribute to and perpetuate oral breathing. Restorative breathing and Buteyko methods are some that are employed. Correcting the volume and rate of breathing can help reduce the collapse of the airway passages. Nasal breathing is a requirement in correction of an OMD.

When I received training from Patrick McKeown to become a Level 3 Buteyko Educator, I had no idea that it would so profoundly impact my own health. I had become trained for my patients but was unaware I was oral breathing while talking all day in my new Myo profession, plus I was snoring with congestion at night. I had struggled with acne, brain fog, headaches, Raynaud's disease, eczema, and fatigue for years, and it was getting worse. Applying Buteyko methods allowed me to correct most of these issues within two months. I personally understand the work it takes to reap the benefits of nasal breathing. I am forever grateful to Patrick for giving me the tools that I utilize daily with my patients and in my own life. I was still, however, waking up at 4:00 a.m., which required an ALF and osteopathy to correct the structural contributors to my fragmented sleep. Thanks to Dr. Bronson and Dr. Turzo, my sleep and my neck have improved tremendously.

I have also found that extra training in cranial nerve integration and reflexes can be foundational and necessary to correct OMD when retained reflexes are present. Birth trauma (can be minimal, i.e. not identified and/or more serious), PTSD, trauma in general, delayed development, lacking meeting developmental milestones, all can be integral in interrupting progression for normal function.

The best known associations for training in orofacial myofunctional therapy are:

- IAOM (International Association of Orofacial Myology)
- AAMS (Academy of Applied Myofunctional Sciences)

These associations have member directories to aid in finding a therapist (see Resources).

The evaluation process with a potential patient

Body posture, gate, facial balance, symmetry occlusion, function, eating, drinking, health history, diet, and school performance are all assessed. Tongue and lip postures are evaluated. I ask about sleep habits, and the quality of sleep. The stop bang, Epworth sleepiness, or pediatric sleep screening questionnaires may be implemented. Snoring, bedwetting, night terrors, and no dreaming may indicate more testing such as sleep studies are in order. It is ideal to get a baseline with these studies prior to therapy and one at the end of treatment if possible, to make sure the symptomatology has been addressed.

Birth histories can be helpful, especially whether and for how long breastfeeding was practiced, and the experience for both the mother and child. Frequency of colds and ear infections, allergies, as well as breathing related problems such as sinusitis, asthma, and chronic rhinitis are indicators that perhaps additional professionals like an osteopath, an ENT, or allergist (as well) as may need to be enlisted for resolution. The patient's functional speech patterning is evaluated and referrals to a speech pathologist are made as needed.

Questions on habits and motivation are included in order to determine whether or not the individual will be a good candidate for OMFT. Because OMFT requires time and commitment, the ability to accommodate OMFT appointments is also addressed. Measurements and assessment photos are taken initially and throughout therapy to track treatment progress and for communication purposes with the patients or other professionals.

Extraoral observations

- Posture, gait
- Facial profile
- Symmetry: body, face, head
- Cervical spine and head position
- Eyes: track, converge, glasses
- Nares: size and responsiveness
- Lips: open versus closed, chapped, flaccid, shorter upper lip, tight with minimal vermillion border, tone
- Allergic shiners, allergic salute (fine line across top of nose from rubbing nose), congestion
- Audible breathing, yawning, sighing, over-breathing
- Visible upper chest breathing, rate, volume
- Eye contact, ability to engage, follow directions, attitude, and parent support
- Hypofunction of the mandibular muscles or hypertrophy of the muscles of mastication. Balance and symmetry noted as well as palpation for tenderness.
- Audible or visual tongue thrust or protrusion of the tongue visible
- Vocal quality changes (chronic hoarseness)
- Excessive contraction of the mentalis

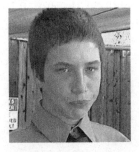

- Facial grimace during a reverse swallow

Intraoral observations

• Oropharyngeal airway: size and depth, color

The Mallampati Score

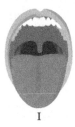 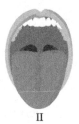 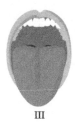 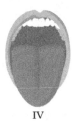

I	II	III	IV
Complete visualization of the soft palate	Complete visualization of the uvula	Visualization of only the base of the uvula	Soft palate is not visible at all

• The tone of the tissue, the narrowness of the airway, and also how much space there is beyond the posterior pillar (curtain) and uvula is important. These images exhibit restricted airways.

Curtains – Oropharyngeal Space

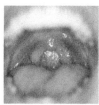 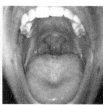 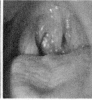

• Tonsils: presence and size and health

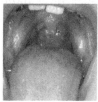 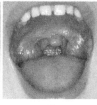 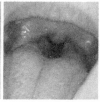 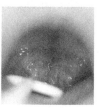

1	2	3	4
Tonsils hidden within tonsil pillars	Tonsils extending to the pillars	Tonsils are beyond the pillars	Tonsils extend to midline

- Tongue surface, shape and size: scalloping, geographic, coated, fissured

- Position of tongue observed during speech

- Position of tongue when mouth is closed and/or at rest, and for the swallow

- Labial, lingual, and buccal frenums: attachment and tension, position, thick, thin, vascularity, submucosal, posterior

- Bruxism, wear patterns, muscular hypertrophy of muscles of mastication and tenderness

- Swallowing (head and cervical motion with a facial grimace may indicate a thrust) anterior, bilateral, unilateral, mandibular, bi-maxillary

- Chewing patterns: lips open, burping, washing food down

- Occlusion: Class I, Class II or Class III malocclusion, cross-bites, open bites, missing teeth, implants, previous orthodontics, iatrogenic dentistry, excessive wear due to bruxism, gingival health, oral hygiene (also an indicator on how compliant the patient will be), anterior teeth with gingivitis and may be mouth breathing

- Is the optimal freeway space (2-3 mm between the molars and 3-5 mm between the incisors) present?

- Size and shape and color of palate, tori present (bony growth due to excessive suction from sleep disordered breathing and/or clenching), height

- Excessive and prominent rugae due to no tongue to palate contact

- Erosion on teeth indicating possible reflux

- Are abfractions (notches on the cervical neck of the tooth from excessive clenching and bruxing) present and how severe?

- History of temporomandibular dysfunction, clicking, popping, previous subluxations, tinnitus, excessive wax, tender to palpitations, trauma

- Habits: thumb/finger sucking, tongue sucking (tongue, cheeks, shirts, objects), and lip, nail biting, leaning, cheek chewing

- Engagement and motivation are customized for that particular patient's age and environmental influences and support

How should a hygienist evaluate OMDs?

There are a number of quick chairside evaluations that may identify a potential OMD. Dental hygienists are in an ideal position to make a number of observations during the extra- and intra-oral exam that should be included in the individual treatment plan so that appropriate care considerations and referrals can be made. Speech pathologists are also in an ideal position to identify OMDs.

Who should be treated?

I begin educating/encouraging youngsters (about nutrition and being active), teenagers (with information about nutrition, avoidance of toxins, as well as posture), and those that are of reproductive age (regarding nutrition, prenatal, breastfeeding, and optimal deliveries if possible). I implore them to take care of their "castles." In order to have healthy offspring these practices are essential for the best outcomes. So, education and prevention are part of treating OMDs.

Infants are encouraged to nurse, and frenula and reflexes evaluated. If facial dysmorphology is suspected, the appropriate professionals should evaluate the use of osteopathy, International Board Certified Lactation Consultants (IBCLC's), as well as possible frenum revisions and body work done before releases. Fascial strain patterns may be "upstream or downstream" with the tongue being the terminal end. For the best outcomes, it is best to "normalize/unwind the strains" of all the tissues along the deep anterior fascial train that goes from the toes to the tongue. The parents are educated with the pre- and post-op exercises, bodywork afterwards will also be necessary, and an OMFT may be part of that team. (This applies to older children and adults as well.) There are orofacial myofunctional therapists and speech pathologists that specialize in babies and can be very helpful in correcting problems early. The sooner oral dysfunction is identified, the sooner the suboptimal craniofacial dysmorphology that follows the emerging OMD may be avoided and/or corrected. There are oral motor exercises as well as feeding interventions appropriate for all ages. Standard myofunctional therapy requires the ability to engage in exercises, but play and games can be integrated and "growing into" phases of myofunctional therapy can be implemented. From cradle to grave OMFT may be beneficial if dysfunction is present.

Benefits of OMFT

Bringing harmony to the function of the muscles can:

- If caught early enough, prevent craniofacial facial dysmorphism and malocclusion that may lead to other comorbidities.

- Guide the teeth into a more desirable relationship during the growth and development years.

- Assist the functional dentist and or orthodontist in his/her attempt to align the teeth and jaws properly.

- Assist in stabilizing the teeth, jaws and functions, during and/or after orthodontic/orthopedic treatment and/or surgery.

- Enhance overall appearance. Resting with the lips together has a positive, cosmetic effect.

- Help stabilize osteopathic/craniosacral adjustments/physical therapy.

- Promote better head and neck posture.

- Reduce periodontal problems due to mouth breathing and thrusting against teeth.

- Help with TMD-related problems as they relate to the musculature, habits, functions and postures.

- Improve digestive problems due to inappropriate chewing and swallowing patterns as well as table manners.

- Aid in achieving nasal breathing as the dominant respiratory function with a relaxed lip seal.

Acknowledgments

I owe an abundance of gratitude to all of the many mentors that have educated, inspired, and guided me. My father was a dentist with a progressive practice 45+ years ago. He encouraged his then hygienist Joy Moller, RDH, to train in OMFT to deliver orofacial myofunctional therapy and nutritional counseling in his office where he also aided patients with TMD and preventive dentistry. In 2004 I had the blessing to intern and study myofunctional therapy with the AOMT team of Joy Moeller, RDH, and Barbara Greene; and later with some of the pioneers of OMFT: the Zickefooses, Sandra Coulson, and Kim Benkert, RDH. I received my Certification of Orofacial Myofunctional therapy (COM™) from the IAOM in 2010. The AAMS (who provide training/AOMT) and the IAOM have provided yearly conferences that I religiously attend, as well as AAPMD. I received training from Patrick McKeown and Robert Litman workshops for Buteyko and the BBEA has supportive conferences as well. The ability to deal with conversion to nasal breathing with the aid of these modalities was a game changer for my practice because I could actually get mouth breathers to habituate to proper oral postures once the breathing was addressed. Svetlana Masgatova for MNRI, Lois Layne for cranial nerve and restorative breathing, and Maxine Haller, OT, for further cranial nerve reflexes have been an invaluable part of the armamentarium that I've added to my practice. Darick Nordstrom, DDS, James Bronson, DDS, and Randolph Miller, DMD, have been my ALF mentors. Dr. Tasha Turzo has so graciously introduced me to the world of osteopathy and the positive impact it can have on lives. I am forever grateful to you all.

CHAPTER 5

Postural Changes and Malocclusions

Head forward posture syndrome

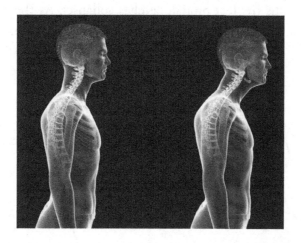

The above image shows the head positioned forward over the cervical vertebrae.

When I began my practice in 1996, the diagnosis of Head Forward Posture Syndrome (HFP) did not exist. Now, it is known as the most common postural syndrome. Basically, it is a posture where the head is forward over the neck and shoulders and creates a structural shift in the vertebral alignment and pelvic rotation downstream to the feet. It's a syndrome that creates more symptoms and is also known as "scholar's neck," "text neck" and "reading neck."

For many reasons that I will examine in this chapter, the head moves anteriorly (forward) on the atlas (first cervical vertebra) shifting the body's center of gravity forward. For every inch of forward motion of the head, the neck experiences an increased load of 10 lbs.! The increased pressure on the cervical vertebrae increases the risk for arthritis and herniated discs. The change in gravity also affects all the curves of the spine with an increase in cervical lordosis, thoracic kyphosis, and lumbar lordosis. The normal curves of the spine are exaggerated in curvature. The pelvis rotates downwards (anteriorly), which internally rotates the head of the femur and thus the feet pronate (arches collapse). As the head moves forward, the shoulders also fall forward and the shoulder blades "wing" outwards.

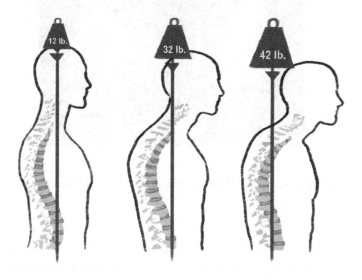

As the head moves forward in relation to the cervical spine, the increase in load is 10 lbs. for every inch of forward displacement of the head.

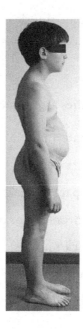

This image shows a head forward posture, forward rolling of the shoulders, and forward tilt of the pelvis and the feet collapse inward.[1]

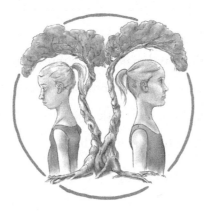

The above picture depicts the upper body's response to HFP. The head is forward, eyes have a downward gaze, the mandible is back (which limits room for the tongue) so there is a "bulge" of tissue under the mandible where the tongue is laying low, the shoulders are forward, and the scapula (shoulder blades) are "winged." The HFP is also created by open mouth posture, chronic sinusitis and/or allergies, tongue-ties, temporomandibular dysfunction (TMD), and airways restrictions (more to be discussed below).

Muscles involved in the postures associated with head forward posture:

The front neck muscles elongate and weaken:

- Longus colli (front part of neck)
- Longus capitis (front part of neck)
- Infrahyoid and suprahyoid (front part of neck)
- Rhomboids (upper back muscles)
- Serratus anterior (along the side of the ribs)
- Lower trapezius (mid back)

The back neck muscles become shorter and tighter:

- Suboccipitals (base of the skull)
- Sternocleidomastoid (side and front of neck)
- Upper trapezius (upper back)
- Pectoralis minor and major (chest muscles)
- Levator scapulae (neck down to shoulder blade)
- Subscapularis (shoulder blade area)
- Latissimus dorsi (mid to lower back)

Symptoms of head forward posture include:

- Muscle tightness
- Kyphosis (excessive rounded shoulders)
- Neck tightness/pain
- Back pain
- Muscle spasms

- Restricted breathing
- Headaches and migraines
- Insomnia
- Sleep apnea
- Chronic fatigue
- Numbness and tingling of the arms and hands
- Temporomandibular joint (TMJ) pain

Habits and conditions that contribute to head forward posture include:

- Extended computer use with poor ergonomics
- Extended cell phone use ("text neck")
- Car seats and strollers with "C" shape for infants/toddlers
- Car seats for adults with headrests that bring head forward
- Open mouth breathing and posturing
- Anterior tongue thrust
- Myofunctional dysfunctions
- Airway and breathing dysfunctions
- Carrying heavy backpacks
- Allergies
- History of cervical whiplash injury
- "Gaming" in slouched positions
- Too much back support since birth

Basic test for head forward posture

1. Stand with your back towards a wall with your heels positioned shoulder width apart and parallel with each other.

2. Press your buttocks against the wall and make sure that your shoulder blades are in contact with the wall.

3. Squeeze your shoulder blades together to get your shoulders into a more neutral position and,

4. If in this position your head is not able to rest against the wall then you have head forward posture (image on right).

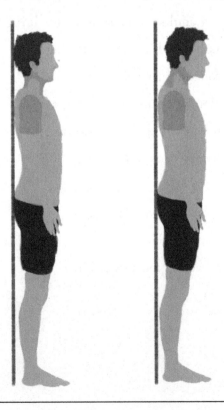

Causes of head forward posture syndrome

The simple explanation for head forward posture is poor posture habits, or slouching. The habit of sitting or standing without engaging core abdominal muscles will lead to a head forward posture. So, any activity that is happening without core activation is termed "bad posture." I have found yoga, Pilates, and/or working with a personal trainer who is educated in functional core rehabilitation to be extremely helpful for my patients and myself to relearn how to move from the core.

Another etiology which can create this posture begins with the baby's first car ride. Our infant seats and strollers are mostly "C" shaped. The baby is curled into a "C" position with its head placed forward and the upper and lower back rounding. I have treated many children who have rounded backs due to prolonged time in car seats and strollers. This tends to happen to the little ones that don't sleep well and whose parents drive them all around town trying to get their kid to sleep. I was one of those moms, too, so no guilt! We do the best we can given what we know at the time. And, yes, both my kids have had many osteopathic treatments to help them grow into their potential and are doing great in life! Interestingly, most car seats, not just the infant car seats, are "C" shaped. You may notice that your head is in a more forward position in your car than when you are just standing. I've had patients buy very "expense top of the line" cars and within several weeks experience new onset headaches and neck pain. The osteopathic treatments could not change the tissue with the constant influence of the car seat creating bad posture. It's best to have a supportive car seat that supports the head alignment on the neck as opposed to a head forward posture. A disengagement of the abdominal core muscles occurs as the lower back rounds and the abdominal muscles shorten and are inhibited. When a baby grows in relation to the shape of the car seat and/or stroller, the very important core muscles are not engaging and activating to create an easeful experience in moving as an upright human being. There are alternative car seats that keep the infant and child in an upright position. One such company is Clek.

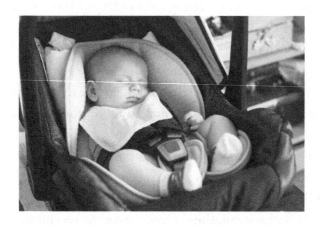

This image shows the typical "C" shape of infant car seats. The back is rounded, which brings the head forward. The rounded back posture shortens and inhibits the abdominal muscles, which are the core muscles needed for upright posture.

The "holding" and "prompting" devices we have are inhibiting our children's neuromuscular skeletal development. When our baby is learning to turn over, we see it struggle over and over to make that move. It's the effort that is building neuromuscular skeletal pathways and forming capacities. As parents we do not want to interfere in any way with this perfect unfolding of the neuromuscular skeletal system that is being stimulated by this effort. Allow the effort to happen within a safe environment. I have found this perception to be pivotal as a parent in all the development stages of raising children even into parenting adult children. Allow the children to make their own efforts with their own initiation within their current developmental stage. This is the foundation for creating self-confidence.

So, if your child cannot sit up on its own, then it is not beneficial from a neuromuscular skeletal viewpoint to be "propped" up in a seating position for long periods of time. If the infant is unable to stand on its own, then the neurodevelopment integration is not able to engage all the complexities needed for upright stance without compensations, which can include a disruption of the core engagement. Other muscles will be used to engage visual and vestibular balance by over-recruiting the muscles of the spine. These children come into the office with tight upper and lower back muscles and an arching backwards. The anterior abdominal muscles are turned off. When these kids start to walk, they arch their backs, have a wide stance, and hold their arms far away from the midline. These are early signs of the beginning of life long bad posture habits. So, not only are these propping devices robbing children of physiological neuromuscular integration, they are also taking away an opportunity for children to build the confidence that develops out of the struggle and effort made towards achievement. The achievement is empty without the developmental changes that are created by the process. So, let your child discover their own capacities by providing safe environments for them to make an effort! And, of course, to learn from their mistakes.

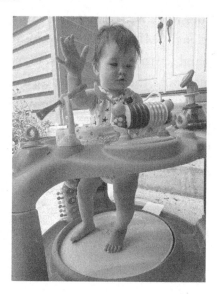

In the late 1990s, cell phones started becoming more mainstream. It's been a head forward downhill postural experience since then. The image below says it all. These days, anywhere we walk a variation of the below posture can be seen. But what is fascinating (at least to me!) is what this posture is doing to the facial growth and development of our children and grandchildren. What is the interplay of forward head posture, malocclusions, myofunctional dysfunctions, tongue-ties, and TMD?

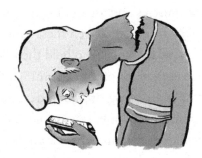

The above image is an all too common posture for most of us.

Most of the practitioners working in the field of neuromuscular medicine regard HFP as a postural change secondary to poor posture habits. The complexity comes when we connect the postural patterns of myofunctional dysfunctions, TMD, the dental occlusion, sleep apnea, and breathing disorders and see that the head forward posture is a compensation in order to maximize the space at the back of the tongue called our "airway." That is not to say that all people with HFP syndrome would benefit from the exercises given to strengthen their core, back and neck muscles, or seeing an osteopath or Pilates therapist, maintaining a regular yoga practice, changing the bad habits that contribute to this posturing, or being fitted with an ALF appliance. But, people in the neuromuscular skeletal professions need to understand that HFP can be a result of airway deficiency, malocclusions, tongue-ties, TMD, and/or myofunctional dysfunction; and these issues need to be addressed and integrated into health before the postural changes can be sustained in a physiological posture from any exercises or soft tissue adjustments. The body will prioritize survival first, which is airway as well as the dental occlusion for breathing, chewing, and swallowing. This is another great example of how a collaborative approach to working with malocclusions, airway deficiencies, and neuromuscular integration is so vitally potent and important.

The compensations of the entire neuromuscular skeletal system that are activated with head forward posturing include postural neuro-input from the head, jaw, tongue, lips, eyes, vestibular portion of the inner ear, specialized sensory cells, spindles in the muscles; and sensors in the articulation of the joints, skin, fascia and internal organ stretch and feet. The physical expression of the above may look like your child slumped on a couch!

Head position influences the dental occlusion

The mandible and head position are reciprocally related. The mandible began to have an effect on posture when we developed from quadrupeds, where the head and mandible hung off the front of the spine, to an upright human being with our heads and mandibles positioned on top of the cervical spine. When we went from walking on all fours to two feet, our mandibles became important in our postural support. The jaw and postural muscles developed coordinated firing patterns and our skeleton and feet develop curves to absorb and distribute the forces of gravity.[2] [3]

The change in horizontal to a vertical stance also created a change in the pivot point of connection between the cranium and cervical, which was the driving force for a remodeling of the cranial base to have a distinct curve and sharp bend. This allowed the occipital condyles to form a joint with the first cervical vertebra, stabilizing an upright stance with a horizontal visual glaze.[4]

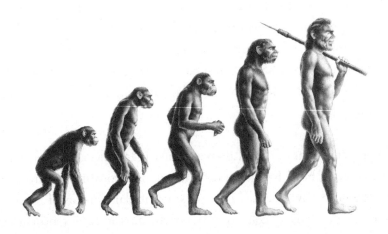

This shift also included a change in the face, which became less elongated and moved posteriorly, compromising our airway space.

The change from walking on all fours to two feet compromised the forward position of our face. As the distance from the back of the neck to the front of the face shortened, so has the space for our airway.

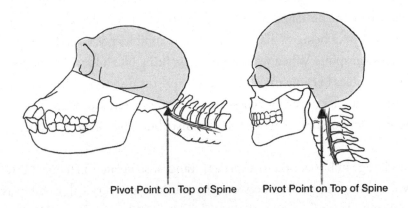

Pivot Point on Top of Spine   Pivot Point on Top of Spine

The cranium was reshaped for upright posture. Notice the increase in angle of the cranium, the shortening of the mandible, and the change of the pivot point connection between the cranium and cervical vertebra. These are the craniofacial cervical adaptations needed for an upright posturing, which allowed humans to use their hands.

The good news is that we had more space for our brains to get bigger, so we got smarter. The bad news is we had less space for our airway and tongue. Thus making breathing and running from lions and tigers more challenging! So, we began to develop tools with our brains and hands to protect ourselves instead of running.

The body is one functional unit with all neuro-immune endocrine musculoskeletal systems interacting in a balancing system of feedback communications. The tongue movement in swallowing, chewing, and the resting posture will affect the teeth position, and how the teeth interdigitate will influence the position of the mandible. The position of the mandible plays a crucial role in the posture of the head on the cervical vertebra, which affects vertebrae and pelvic changes down through to the feet. And, just as the position of the teeth affects the mandible and head positional changes, so does an asymmetrical gait, foot stance, pelvic asymmetry and/or shoulder dysfunction affect mandibular and head position. Changing the mandibular position affects the body posture and conversely, changing the body posture affects the mandibular position. A study showed that placing a heel lift shifted the occlusion to the same side as the placed heel lift.[5] Increasing the height on one leg shifts the pelvis to the opposite side, thus creating the need for the reciprocal sideways movement with the mandible to occur in order to center the head and eyes. One can see here the pattern of scoliosis that can develop from mandibular deviation and having a shorter leg on one side.

If mandibular posture shifts in one direction, the head posture shifts in the opposite direction. The occlusion and body posture are codependent variables. There are many studies that support the interdependence connection between mandibular position and postural changes.[6][7][8]

Any change in one area affects another. I am highlighting malocclusion and TMD as contributors to postural ailments because they are commonly missed by most practitioners working in the field of dentistry and neuromuscular medicine. Because the dental occlusion and TMD are largely misunderstood and overlooked components of postural ailments, and thus often not incorporated into the treatment of musculoskeletal dysfunctions, relapse continues to be an issue. In other words, if the asymmetry in the pelvis is due to TMD, the asymmetry will not integrate until the TMD is treated. The opposite is also true. If the TMD is due to pelvic dysfunction, the pelvis asymmetry will need to be addressed in order to resolve the TMD. It is also important to note that a mandibular splint is not a cure for TMD but instead can be a vital component of a treatment plan for a patient. The cure happens when the patient has a physiological occlusion that supports the health of the joint and alignment of the body, and is no longer splint dependent.[9]

The posterior mandibular posture causes anterior head posture by stimulating changes in posture to protect the airway. The position of the mandible affects and is affected by the volume of the airway. The mandible surrounds the pharynx on three sides and the cervical spine is the fourth border. The posterior displacement of the mandible (backwards position) can diminish the cross-sectional area of the pharyngeal airway. In response to survival needs, all the muscles of the craniofacial cervical complex adapt their resting postures to hold the bones and soft tissue in the positions to maximize airway space. Typically, the head extends backwards in order to rotate the mandible anteriorly and superiorly, which also brings the tongue forward. As the tongue and mandible move away from the cervical spine, the space between, our airway, expands, thereby increasing its distance away from the cervical spine and opening the space behind the tongue. The increase in pharyngeal airway space produced by head extension has been demonstrated with imaging.[10] [11] Also, remember that this space called our "airway" is a collapsible tube of soft tissue whose shape is dependent on the muscle contraction and ligament tone, and the position and shape of the mandible, maxilla, and cervical spine. Of course, the shape, tone, and movement of the tongue will also influence the shape and size of the airway.

However, the head cannot just tip backward, because visual and vestibular reflexes (the so-called righting reflexes) keep it level with the horizon.[12] [13]

As a result of these reflexes, the head can only extend if it also translates anteriorly, which produces the head forward position with the increase in extension of the cervical vertebrae. The mandible can have two postural influences acting to stabilize; one coming from the posturing of the head, neck, tongue and airway influence; and the other from the "uprighting" visual reflex. The two influences need to be integrated for the patient to not have either neck or jaw pain as they may be being influenced by two different postural balancing systems. There are many studies looking at the interplay between the dental occlusion and posture. One study investigated the effect of the following dental malocclusions:

- posterior unilateral crossbites (one side of the upper jaw is positioned inside of the lower jaw)

- bilateral crossbites (both sides of the upper jaw bone is placed inside of the lower jaw bone)

- contraction of the temporalis, sternocleidomastoid, trapezius and cervical muscles

The anterior temporalis on the side of the unilateral cross bite was overactive when the mandible was in a resting position. Bilateral crossbite patients have an increase in electromyography (EMG) activity in their sternocleidomastoid muscles compared to the control group without crossbites.[14] (An EMG is a diagnostic procedure that evaluates the health condition of muscles and the nerve cells that control them.)

After working in collaboration with dentists using functional biocompatible dental appliances since 1996, I have been continuously amazed to feel and see how micro changes in the dental occlusion create movement and positional changes in the craniofacial cervical complex and whole body. For example, the smallest change in a lower mandibular splint changing a tooth contact can create a change to the temporal bones bringing them into balance. There are many studies showing the positional connection between the mandible, head, cervical, and postural connection.[15-34]

As stated in the preface of this book, there is a change in facial growth and development to an increase in Class 2 (upper jaw forward position), and an average change toward a more posterior mandibular posture may be an important cause of the accompanying average change toward a more anterior head posture. In population studies, posterior mandibular posture and anterior head posture are well correlated.[35][36] Studies also correlate body posture and mandibular growth.[37][38] Chapter 8 goes into this subject in more detail.

There is a correlation between Class II occlusion (maxilla forward and mandible back), forward head posture, and craniomandibular dysfunction.[39]

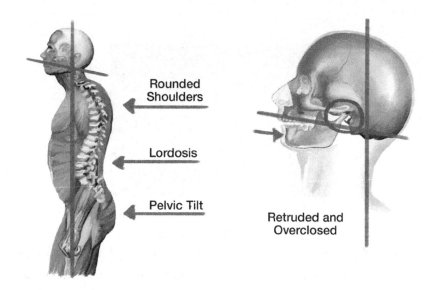

Rounded Shoulders

Lordosis

Pelvic Tilt

Retruded and Overclosed

The above image shows the maxilla and head forward posture with the mandible reflexives moving backwards.

Connection between mandibular lateral displacement and scoliosis

The anterior and posterior position of the mandible has an effect on the body posture as discussed above. A sideways, lateral displacement of the mandible is associated with rotations and sidebending of the vertebra. A lateral displacement of the mandible can be approximated by comparing the midlines between maxillary and mandibular frena, and has been correlated with scoliosis and other postural asymmetries.[40] [41] [42]

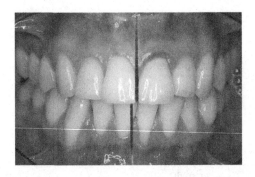

Observe the alignment between the upper and lower maxillary frenulum which can indicate a mandibular shift indicating TMD. The above image is within a normal range of asymmetry and is most likely not clinically relevant.

Studies of healthy subjects have shown that asymmetric occlusal interferences (malocclusions) produce asymmetric firing of neck muscles.[43] As the cervical muscles fire asymmetrically, the vertebrae are pulled out of alignment, creating a twist in the neck. Compensations in body posture can create scoliosis. The younger the age when the malocclusion creates a lateralization of the mandible that stimulates asymmetrical contraction of the cervical muscles, the more compensation the person will have throughout their body and the more difficult it will be to treat the twists. Facial asymmetry has been found to be correlated with shoulder imbalance and adolescent idiopathic scoliosis,[44] lateral displacement of the cervical spine,[45] [46] and increased body sway.[47]

Here is a crucial point. If a mandibular displacement occurs in a child, the body will grow to accommodate the non-physiological position of the mandible. There may be a mild scoliosis as a consequence of the dental occlusion. If traditional orthodontics (heavy wires, high force, short treatment time) reposition the teeth to a midline alignment (forcing teeth into a Class 1 occlusion), the scoliotic pattern is not able to unwind and realign itself to the upper and lower jaws' midline reposition. This leaves the overall somatic experience with more compensations and thus more energy output, which increases the overall sympathetic tone, leaving the person in an autonomic unbalanced and compromised state. When the occlusion has been changed without treating the tissue compensations, the dental occlusion can "lock in" the tissue dysfunctions through the rest of the body. If the teeth position is changed without unwinding the rest of the body for an integrative experience, the strain patterns become very difficult to treat. Every time the teeth are in contact, the strain patterns are reactivated.

How mouth breathing and a dysfunctional swallow creates postural changes

As the mouth opens, the mandibular condyles rotate anteriorly and inferiorly, which brings the head into a flexed position (forward on the spine). The head tilts up as the need for the eyes to be horizontal to the ground stimulates a neuro reflex, which activates and extends the cervical muscles to stabilize the head's anterior movement leading to cervical and spinal changes on down the body. The shoulder blades move forward with the shoulders, and the chain of muscles transmits changes in compensation all the way down to the feet. The connection between a pharyngeal airway blockage that creates head extension and forward head posture can be inferred from findings that most children with swollen tonsils that block their airway have extended head posture. This condition normalizes quickly after a tonsillectomy.[48-51] One study showed that children with nasal respiration age 8 and above present with better posture than those who continue oral breathing beyond age 8.[52]

Any condition that creates open mouth breathing or posturing can stimulate a head forward posture.[53 54] When oral breathing is required for a prolonged period of time, the tongue moves forward to create more space in the airways (obligatory tongue thrust). The tongue is attached to the jaw, so as the tongue moves into a low lying forward resting position it brings the mandible forward.

Many conditions can potentially impair nasal passages. Chronic nasal congestion, whether due to chronic sinusitis or allergies, or a history of asthma, can stimulate an open mouth breathing habit. Physical obstruction of the nasal passages, such as a deviated septum or nasal polyps, could create nasal passage restriction and stimulate an open mouth breathing posture. The most commonly missed causes for chronic nasal obstruction are food allergies. Specifically, dairy is the most common food I have found that creates nasal obstruction. Allergies, whether environmental or food-related, can be the most challenging etiology of chronic nasal obstruction to heal. I start with food elimination diets and food allergy testing to guide the treatment. Toxic mold exposure and Lyme's disease can also create chronic nasal obstruction. A chicken-egg situation is created; as the nasal passageways are congested or blocked, the mouth opens for survival for air, the tongue now rests in the lower jaw, the upper palate collapses without the stimulation by the tongue to widen the palate as the tongue grows, resulting in a discrepancy of palate-to-tongue size. The narrow palate will also be compromised to accommodate the teeth, and thus crowding and malocclusions ensue. The open mouth posture with both low tongue posture and mandible backward will bring the head into a head forward posture. All these changes could be created because of allergies or a dairy sensitivity in a child.

We know that the tongue has many functions including playing a role in speech, chewing, and swallowing. The resting position of the tongue in the palate is the primary stimulation for midface growth and development and provides stabilization for the cranial base as well as augmenting cranial motion. During swallow, the upward pressure of the tongue into the hard and soft palate drains the sinuses and middle ear, and augments the cranial rhythmic movement by increasing motion at the sphenobasilar symphysis. The tongue will also provide stability for an injured temporomandibular joint by thrusting to the affected upper or lower jaw. We know that the tongue is intimately connected to the hyoid, mandible, and temporal bones through muscles and ligaments. So as the tongue goes through its dynamic movements the hyoid, mandible, and cranium adapt and accommodate to the tongue's dynamic movements.

We can think of the tongue as a "rudder" for postural changes. A rudder is the steering device on boats that guides and holds the course. It leads the boat in the desired direction. When the tongue moves forward during an anterior tongue thrust (immature swallow) the head and mandible follow. When the tongue thrusts to the side (laterally) to stabilize TMD the cervical vertebrae rotate to the same side following the tongue. When the tongue is resting in a low posture in the mandible, the head nods forward following the posture of the tongue.

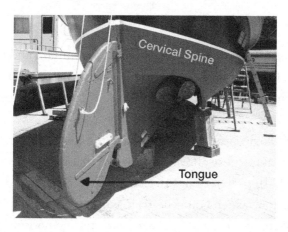

The above image names the rudder of the boat as the tongue and the boat as the cervical spine. A tongue thrust to the right side of the palate will create a rotation of the upper cervical vertebrae, also to the right. We see asymmetrical formation of the palate with ankyloglossia (tongue-tie). As the tongue is restricted in its range of motion during a swallow, one side of the tongue reaches further to the palate, thus creating a wider palate on one side. This asymmetrical contraction and formation of the palate rotates the upper cervical to the side.

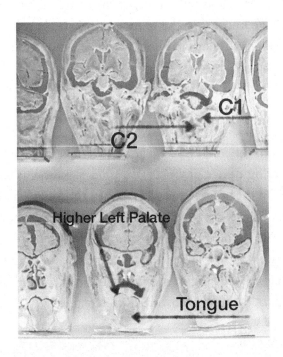

This is an image of a cross section through the cranium and upper cervical vertebra. One can see the position of the tongue is higher in the left palate and the 2nd cervical vertebra is also rotated to the right.

A study by Fabio Scoppa in 2004 presented the glosso-postural syndrome, which linked atypical swallows with postural changes occurring in the entire body.[55] This chapter has presented the relationship between the dental occlusion, which could be seen as the largest joint in the body, and postural changes created by the tongue's resting position and motion during swallow. Scoppa presented common and less common postural changes associated with atypical deglutition (swallow).

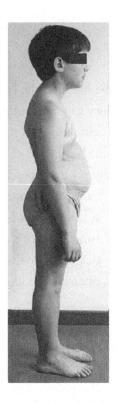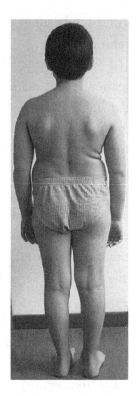

The above images depict the most common posture associated with an anterior thrust dysfunction. We see a forward head posture, mandible forward with tongue thrust and anterior open bite, rounded shoulders, scapular plane in front of the gluteal plane, abdominal muscles hypotonia, and pronated feet.[56]

The tongue can influence the position of the head on the neck and the jaw in the head, but what effect does that have downstream on the rest of the body? The pattern of the tongue during swallow directly affects the movement of the hyoid, and this holds true as the hyoid affects the range of motion for the tongue. As the hyoid has 12 muscles that attach to each side of the hyoid and the hyoid is the only bone in the body that is not attached to another bone but is "floating" in the soft tissue matrix, it can adapt to multiple influences. The hyoid is an "integrator" or "mediator" between the many functions of the tongue and mandible.

The glosso-postural syndrome is characterized by postural imbalance and atypical deglutition.

Besides forming the size and shape of the maxilla, the tongue also participates in a balancing and a compensatory function acting as a stabilizing "joint" in the body supporting the dental occlusion. The tongue is capable of perturbing postural balance due both to its connections with the key anatomical structures and for neurophysiological reasons. The hyoglossus apparatus that links to the maxilla, the skull, the cervical vertebrae and the scapula, the pharynx and the larynx is the true "trait d'union" between the oral and postural functions for the body. Just as atypical deglutition can be considered a cause of malocclusion, so in malocclusions, the tongue can serve as an occasional stabilizing function.

Another interesting study looked at children from the ages of 7-11 years old radiologically (by X-rays) with atypical swallowing patterns to identify asymmetry in the occipitocervical (the joint that connects the base of the head and the first cervical vertebra) region.[57] The results showed an increase in space between the base of the head and the first cervical vertebra. As we discussed above, as the head rotates backwards (posteriorly) the head moves forward as a postural compensation to keep the eyes horizontal to the ground and thus allowing upright balancing to occur. This connects atypical swallowing with cervical repositioning for postural balance.

This study radiologically identified 352 children with asymmetry in the occipitocervical region and these children were assessed on a number of myofunctional measures.[58] In all children an orthopedic examination was conducted including a functional test of the upper cervical spine and the iliac joint (the joint between the sacrum and ilium), the postural test, as well as gait analysis. The orofacial myofunctional status was evaluated. About 70% of the children revealed orofacial myofunctional disorders. A weak body posture was associated significantly with all myofunctional dysfunctions found. The head was also noted to be reclined (posteriorly rotated) with myofunctional dysfunctions. A restriction of the ilium (pelvic bone) correlated significantly with tongue dysfunction, whereas asymmetry of the upper cervical spine correlated significantly with open mouth posturing. This study points to the importance of diagnosing and treating the entire body when addressing myofunctional dysfunctions and malocclusions and the importance of early interdisciplinary screening in children to ensure a physiological development of the orofacial regions and the growing vertebral column.

It is clear that a myofunctional dysfunction defined as an abnormal movement of the tongue can create malocclusion by applying pressure to teeth, moving them out of "alignment." As the tongue is the rudder for the upper cervical vertebra, a conclusion can be made that malocclusion is associated with misaligned upper cervical (neck) vertebrae. This brings to our attention the importance of treating the misaligned vertebrae in relationship with treating the malocclusions. Over the years of my practice I have seen damage to the ligaments and tendons that support the integrity and support of the cervical vertebrae caused by forced adjustment (the "snap, crackle and pop" adjustments) in an attempt to re-align the vertebrae, which are quickly pulled out of alignment by the patient's next abnormal swallowing pattern. These are the patients for which I have needed to re-stabilize the damaged ligaments and tendons, which are made of collagen and fascia, with prolotherapy and/or PRP (Plasma Rich Platelet) therapy. These are also the patients who present with chronic pain syndromes. The collaborative approach with the ALF, myofunctional therapist, and a cranial osteopath can usually address all the components of the craniofacial cervical complex.

CHAPTER 6

The Temporomandibular Joint: An Integrated Perspective

Introduction of temporomandibular dysfunction

The temporomandibular joint (TMJ) is crucial in balancing the cranio-cervical mandibular dental complex, but we still have much to learn about its contribution to craniofacial dysfunction, vagal dysfunctions, neurodegenerative diseases, glymphatics, airway dysfunction, and movement disorders, as well as diffuse and localized chronic pain syndromes.

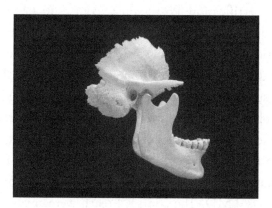

The TMJ connects the temporal bone to the mandible. This joint also connects the cranium to the face.

The mandible is an exceptionally unique bone and its growth and development depends on a multitude of complex influences. These are essential to give the condyle and ramus the growth capacity and adaptability to optimize the essential life functions of breathing, chewing, eating, and swallowing, as well as the important functions such as speaking, standing, sitting, and walking. There is no function in the body that does not have a direct or indirect effect on mandibular growth. The most essential functions of the mandible are to provide nutrition to the body through chewing and swallowing as well as support the soft tissue collapsible tube called our airway for breathing. The mandible is the most important life-giving supportive bone in our body. There are many influences on its growth and development which allow for the adaptability needed to survive with optimal health.

Who is a temporomandibular disorder specialist?

Unfortunately, there is no one particular area of medicine or dentistry that has a board certification to qualify someone as an expert in treating temporomandibular dysfunction (TMD). Any dentist or physician can advertise that they are a specialist in treating TMD without any regulations or certification. Postgraduate courses in TMD are available for both the dentist (DDS) and physician (DO/MD) but there are no board regulations for standard of care treatment. Oral and maxillofacial surgeons are dentists, some of whom also have a medical degree, who specialize in surgical procedures. Osteopathic physicians practicing in the specialty of neuromuscular medicine have minimal formal education in assessing the influences either of the dental occlusion or the soft tissue influences on the dental occlusion. We are taught basic treatments for TMD but many of my colleagues have no training in how the dental occlusion affects TMD. The courses I teach were created to provide a unified curriculum to bridge the gaps within the dental, osteopathic, and myofunctional therapist education of the interplay between the effect of a dental occlusion and the neuromuscular skeletal system.

The dental occlusion can be considered the maxillary mandibular suture and is the largest joint in the body. It stabilizes the cranial base and can be thought of as a "cranial suture." The motion within the TMJ is essential to assess and learn to treat as it connects the dental occlusion to the face, the cranium, spine, pelvis, and on down to the feet. Many of the dentists practicing as a TMD specialist have minimal to no education in the importance of the soft tissue influences and craniofacial movement on the health of the joint. Dentists have no formal education in assessing the motion and position of the bones of the cranium. The focus for the dentist working with TMD is to change the dental occlusion, usually with splint therapy. This changes the position and location of the mandibular condyle in the temporal mandibular fossa as well as the attachment and functioning of the muscles of mastication. In some cases this can be very helpful. Learning to assess the position and motion of the temporal bone and cranium, as well as looking at the postural compromises, is what is missing in the dentist's education.

A cranial-trained osteopath can assess the motion and position of the temporal bone but is not formally trained to assess how the dental occlusion affects the motion and position of the temporal bone, as well as all the bones in the craniofacial complex and down to the feet. Thus the diagnosis and treatment of the TMJ which provides an essential life stability to our airway and nutrition falls into a large "crack" about the size of the Grand Canyon in our medical dental professions. What is astounding is that 10 million people suffer from TMD with a prevalence in females in the 18-45 years old age range (our estrogen time!). A collaborative approach to treating TMD is essential to provide optimal care for our patients. Dentists trained to assess the motion and position of the temporal bone and osteopaths who learn how to integrate malocclusion into their assessment and treatment of their patients will be providing optimal care for our TMD patients.

Anatomy and the unique features of the TMJ

The TMJ is a ginglymoarthrodial joint, which can have both rotational and translational movements. The initial movement of the condyle is a rotation that occurs in the lower joint space, after which a translation occurs in the superior joint space. Both of these movements must move easily to maintain the health of the joint. The TMJ is formed by the mandibular condyle fitting into the mandibular fossa of the temporal bone with an articular disc, which is suspended by four ligaments attaching to the mandible and the temporal bones. Interestingly, the disc is composed of dense fibrous connective tissue and has no nerve innervation or blood supply, relying solely for its nutrients from the intra articular synovial fluid and compression forces into the joint (chewing) that drive the nutrients into the disc. The posterior ligament that attaches the disc to the mandibular fossa is also called the retrodiscal tissue and is richly vascularized and innervated.[1]

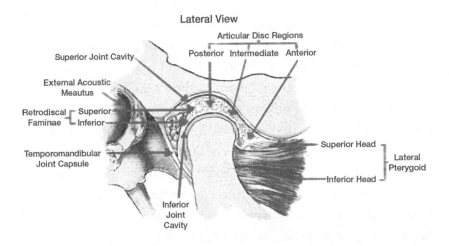

This image indicates the complex anatomy of the TMJ. The retrodiscal tissues are vulnerable to tears resulting from over-contractions or muscle spasms of the superior head of the lateral pterygoid muscle.

One cause of TMD occurs when there are tears or injuries to the posterior ligament (retrodiscal tissue), which becomes overstretched or torn in an attempt to stabilize the disc's physiological position on the mandibular condyle due to an overly contracted muscle which attaches onto the front of the disc. This situation can occur during a whiplash injury to the neck and head, as in a car accident, or with any head injury. The anterior disc attaches to the joint capsule and the superior head of the lateral pterygoid muscle. In whiplash injuries the lateral pterygoid muscle, attached to the front of the disc, goes into spasm and pulls the disc forward and out of position. Its fibers are overstretched in an attempt to stabilize the whiplash. This also occurs to the mandible, which is suspended from the temporal, sphenoid, and hyoid bones by ligaments and muscles. A similar situation can occur with prolonged open mouth posturing in the dental chair. The lateral pterygoid muscle fibers over-contract, pulling the disc forward, creating pain in the jaw joint and causing an inability to either open or close the mouth secondary to the displaced TMJ disc (see 'Etiologies of TMD'). Many dentists will treat with a splint or suggest surgery. Intra oral osteopathic treatments can reposition the disc and restore physiological motion of the jaw joint[2] by releasing the over contracted lateral pterygoid muscles.

Because the TMJ is different in composition and development from other joints in the body there are certain diseases that affect every joint in the body except for the TMJ, and conversely certain diseases that target the TMJ. The articular surface of the mandible is quite complex with four different tissue layers, each having a specific responsibility for stimulation or retardation of growth as well as providing lubrication for ease of motion in the joint. These tissues have receptors for hormones, vitamin D, thyroid, and proteins. Again we see the unique complexity in this joint expressing its need for adaptability for survival. It's our joint for our airway and nourishment! The TMJ is also different because it is composed of fibrocartilage on the mandibular condyle and hyaline cartilage in the temporal fossa.[3] In other synovial joints in the body, the articular surfaces are covered by hyaline cartilage. Fibrocartilage is a tissue with tightly packed cells that create strength for resilience to compressive forces and shearing forces better than hyaline cartilage, making it a superior material for enduring the large amount of occlusal load that is placed on the TMJ.[4] These tightly packed fibrocartilage cells are able to withstand the forces of movement, less susceptible to the effects of aging, less likely to break down over time, and have a better ability to repair themselves.[5]

The unique fibrocartilage on the mandibular condyle has receptors to estrogen and progesterone, which may explain the high prevalence of TMD in reproductive age women.[6]

It has been postulated that the hormonal influences from estrogen, progesterone, and relaxin, may make an individual susceptible to degenerative TMJ diseases. Several lines of evidence support this hypothesis. Both estrogen and progesterone receptors have been localized in the TMJ of human and non-human primates,[7][8][9] in male rats,[10] and in mice of both genders[11] with some findings suggesting a sexual dimorphism in the presence of estrogen receptors.[12]

Other evidence that estrogen is involved in TMDs includes an association between facial pain and estrogen replacement therapy or the use of oral contraceptives,[13][14] and elevated systemic levels of estrogen in women with TMJ disease versus those in normal controls.[15]

Interestingly, estrogen and relaxin may contribute to TMJ degeneration by enhancing the expression of tissue-degrading enzymes belonging to the matrix metalloproteinase (MMP) family that have receptors in TMJ fibrocartilage. MMPs can degrade the collagen and proteoglycans of the cartilage. The studies showed that relaxin and/or estrogen induce specific MMPs, suggesting a plausible role of these enzymes in hormone-mediated joint degeneration. These findings, together with the elevated levels of estrogen in women with TMJ disease, suggest specific sex hormones play a role in causing or predisposing to TMJ degeneration.

Another correlation between TMD and sex hormones was in a study that showed 26 of the 27 women with severe condylar resorption had either laboratory findings of low 17 beta-estradiol or a history of extremely irregular menstrual cycles. Of the 27 women, 25 showed abnormally low levels of serum 17 beta-estradiol at midcycle. These women subsequently experienced a "spontaneous" open bite within six months of taking the birth control pill, also creating a low mid cycle estrogen level and an increase in mandibular condylar resorption.[16]

During my Osteopathic Teaching Fellowship, I had the honor of receiving a Burroughs Wellcome Fellowship in 1993 to research the micro articular surface of the sacroiliac joint. I was able to slice cadaver sacroiliac joints into 1-2 mm sections, and using AutoCAD software, scan the sections to create a 3-D image of the joint, which could be used to create movement animations to study the biomechanics of the joint. The sacroiliac joint is another incredibly unique joint much like the TMJ. These joints are unique in that they are bilateral joints that function as one unit. Since the TMJ is connected to the mandible, the right and left joints must function together and are not independent of each other. This is also true for the sacroiliac joint. Each joint is individually shaped. The sacroiliac joint is like a fingerprint as the interdigitations of the "valleys" and "peaks" on the surface are unique to each individual joint. The adaptability of growth in the TMJ also means that each joint can be quite different in their features, even between right and left. Although all joints can exhibit individual variations to some degree from person to person, the degree of variation seems to be greatest in the mandible, sacrum, and ilium articular surfaces. Also, it's quite interesting that the TMJ and the SI are located in the same vertical plane in the body. I'm curious about that, too.

Symptoms of TMD

Symptoms of TMD include:

- Articular noises: clicking, crepitation in the joint with opening and closing the jaw

- Otic (ear) complaints such as tinnitus, sensation of blockage, and sensations of exaggerated or diminished hearing

- Ocular (eye) disturbance such as peri- or retro-orbital discomfort, excessive lacrimation and problems of accommodation (focus)

- Pain or tenderness in the jaw, especially at the area of the joint

- Popping/clicking of the jaw (crepitus)

- Pain that feels like a toothache (phantom tooth pain)

- Ear pain (earache) or sounds of cracking in the ears

- Ringing or popping sounds in the ears (tinnitus) or a sense of fullness in the ears

- Headaches, including migraines

- Blurred vision

- Tight, stiff, or sore jaw or neck muscles

- Muscle spasms in the jaw

- Facial pain, mouth pain, jaw pain, cheek pain, or chin numbness or tingling

- Pain at the base of the tongue

- Pain, swelling, or a lump in the temple area

- Difficulty chewing

- Shoulder pain

- Locking or dislocation of the jaw (usually after widely yawning), referred to as lockjaw

- Dizziness or vertigo

- Difficulty chewing and swallowing
- limited jaw opening (less than 40 mm or three finger height opening)
- Blocked Eustachian tubes (stuffy ears)
- Hearing changes
- Chronic neck and postural tension
- Facial twitches and tics or numbness in the face
- Anomalies of mandibular movement; any side to side movements during chewing or speech

Etiologies of TMD

Etiologies of TMD include:

- Trauma to the head or face
- Whiplash to the body especially affecting the craniofacial cervical complex
- Retained anterior tongue thrust created by prolonged bottle-feeding, nursing and digit sucking
- Ankyloglossia
- Torticollis
- Cross bites
- Open mouth breathing postures
- Facial growth dysfunctions
- Side or stomach sleeping positions
- Biting the nails
- Bruxism/clenching
- Prolonged stress creating overactive muscles of mastication
- Obstructive sleep apnea (both causes TMD and is caused by TMD)

- Hyper flexible conditions
- Lyme's disease
- Toxic mold disease
- Birth control with estrogen dominance and low mid cycle 17 beta estrogen
- Malocclusion
- Prolonged soft diets with poor nutrition
- Myofunctional dysfunctions
- Traditional retractile orthodontics (i.e. braces)
- Traumatic dental extractions
- Maxillary mandibular advancement surgeries
- Pelvic somatic dysfunctions
- Leg length discrepancies
- Flat feet
- Unstable ankle, secondary to history of an ankle injury
- Recurrent ankle sprains with ankle instability
- Sacroiliac instability
- Hormone deficiencies
- Biochemical imbalances (especially low magnesium)

As one can see from the above list of etiologies, TMD is multifactorial. Some causes include injuries to the craniofacial cervical complex, overuse repetitive injuries, nutritional deficiencies, spinal, pelvis and/or feet somatic instability, temporal bone dysfunctions, imbalanced dental occlusion loading, vitamin and hormone deficiencies/imbalances, myofunctional dysfunctions, as well as poor postural habits.

Mechanical overloading, like a repetitive injury, is a commonly missed etiology. The adaptive capacity for the human to move in an upright position requires an intricate neuro integrated feedback system within the craniofacial cervical complex (as well as spinal, pelvic and feet muscles), which works to keep the eyes horizontal to the ground creating a balance and upright posture. The neuromuscular skeletal system will compromise where it needs to in order to maintain this vital upright position.

A head-forward posture is vulnerable to increased stress not only in the neck, but the TMJ. When the head and neck move forward in the sagittal plane, the brain's visual proprioceptors cause the occiput to backward-bend on the first cervical vertebra. This remarkable proprioceptive reflex (Law of Righting) will tilt the head back to level the eyes with the horizon even if it means a compromise to the neck and jaw.[17] With the head and neck jutted forward, stabilizing contractive forces develop in the hyoid and digastric muscles. In essence, the brain is trying to accommodate the forward head posture by pulling the head back using the jaw muscles. Unfortunately, the muscles that are accommodating the head forward posture are the muscles that also open the jaw creating excessive stress in the joint. Unbalanced repetitive loading creates trauma to the TMJ potentially leading to arthritis and deficient growth of the mandible.

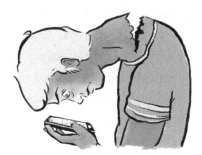

This is an all too common posture which can create overloading in the TMJ.

Studies in mice, rats, rabbits, and non-human primates have shown that normal masticatory function is important for maintaining normal growth, morphology, and function of the cartilage of the TMJ. Most dentists and physicians have been inclined to believe that the single most important etiological factor for degenerative TMJ disease is altered mechanical loading which occurs in malocclusions that surpasses the adaptive capacity of the joint. As practitioners we need to assess our patients' pathology, like TMD, individually and look for their specific cause of dysfunction. When treating TMD, we need to be aware of the vast number of potential causes and develop the necessary tools to treat the causes of and the TMD pathology.

The muscles of mastication and the cranial cervical complex are physiologically neutral when the dental occlusion is stable and balanced, creating a neutral bite. In rodents, altering masticatory loading with a soft diet and/or incisor clipping (cutting down the incisor teeth to change the dental contact) causes structural changes within the condylar cartilage and bone. There was a decrease in the thickness of the mandibular condylar cartilage,[18] [19] [20] a reduction in extracellular cartilage matrix,[21] and a reduction of chondrocyte growth.[22] [23] [24] They found that incisor trimming (discluding the occlusion) and soft diets, creating lack of use of the TMJ causes a transient reversible decrease in the bone volume and trabecular thickness of the mandibular condylar for two to four weeks, which were restored to normal levels over four to six weeks.[25] These changes in the bone by altered TMJ masticatory loading are consistent with changes in the subchondral bone reported for TMJ osteoarthritis. These studies point to the TMJ's incredible capacity for adaptive changes. The change in the bone and cartilaginous growth of the mandible with a change in the diet from soft to hard food was seen over a time frame of weeks. This leads us to believe that the capacity for TMD to heal is more rapid than seen in other joints rehabilitation. When the mandible is not being used, as seen in soft diets, or being used "incorrectly," it does not grow optimally. Basically, if you don't use it you lose it.

The condyle of the mandible is unique in structure. It has a specialized cartilaginous tissue that allows the bone to grow in response to not only the amount of compressive forces through chewing, but also the directional pattern of the chewing. That is to say, the power of contact between the upper and lower teeth and the position of the vector force created by the position of the teeth and position of the condylar process in the fossa will determine the shape and size of the mandibular condyle. This is important to know when we are treating children with facial trauma. The position of the mandibular condyle in the temporomandibular fossa (the joint space) will have a direct effect on the potential growth of the ramus (length) of the mandible.

One may ask the question, why is the mandible so adaptable to usage? For example, soft diets decrease the growth of the mandible and hard foods increase the size. The answer lies in epigenetics, which describes the condition of cellular activity activation that is dependent on the interplay between one's environment and genetics. We are not just an expression of our genes. We are complex beings who are constantly being remodeled to meet the demands of our current conditions. However, the mandible stands out with its capacity for adaptive growth. Why? Because it is the bone that supports our airway, which is essential to life. As we grow, we adapt to optimize our airway just as a plant grows toward sunshine.

Traumatic injuries are also an important etiological factor in the development of TMJ disorders. One study examining 400 consecutive TMD patients found that, in 24.5 percent of patients, the onset of the pain could be linked directly to the trauma.[26] Individuals who have been in automobile accidents and sustained whiplash injuries increase risk of developing TMDs. In recent studies, it has been shown that there is an increase in developing limited or painful jaw movements immediately after whiplash injury[27] and that one in three people who are exposed to whiplash trauma are at risk of developing delayed TMJ symptoms.[28] The mandible is suspended by ligaments and muscles to the sphenoid and temporal bones. Any whiplash that occurs to the cranium and cervical vertebrae (neck) also impacts the mandible. If there is a cervical whiplash the TMJ sustains the same forces of injury. The lateral pterygoid muscle is usually the culprit of TMD caused by whiplash injuries. The muscle is unique in that it has two parts to it, the upper head of the muscle attaches directly onto the front of the TMJ disc and the lower head attaches to the mandible. The over contraction of the upper head of the lateral pterygoid muscle can pull the disc forward thus displacing it from its physiological position on top of the mandibular condyle. This creates a limited capacity to open the jaw and can create pain and clicking when opening and closing the jaw. This condition is not uncommon and requires immediate osteopathic treatment to release the over-contraction of the lateral pterygoid muscle to allow the disc to slip back into place.

A whiplash injury can also occur by falling on one's chin or other part of the face, creating an over-extension of the neck and compression of the mandible. If the force is powerful enough, the mandible could fracture and/or the disc could be misplaced or even torn. The blood supply to the cartilaginous disc is like all the discs in the vertebra, it is reliant on the contraction and elongation of the muscles to literally pump blood into the cartilaginous tissue. For this reason, compromised discs need repair. It is essential to help the muscles regain their capacity to maintain maximum elongation and contraction. The lateral pterygoid muscle is the most important muscle to treat as it attaches directly onto the disc of the TMJ. The growth of the mandible depends on the position of the disc on top of the mandibular condyle. When the disc is in its proper place there is optimal growth stimulation. I have seen many patients with asymmetrical growth of their mandibles as a result of an early childhood trauma that affected the growth and development of the mandible.

Motor vehicle accidents are a common cause of whiplash and injury to the neck and also to the TMJ. Many people have experienced pain, popping, crepitus and/or a change in the opening width of the mouth after a car accident. These symptoms indicate that the lateral pterygoid muscle as well as other muscles in the craniofacial cervical complex are strained and over-contracted. When the lateral pterygoid muscle becomes acutely contracted, there is a potential for the anterior pull on the disc to displace the disc. If the disc is positioned in front of the mandibular condylar, instead of its position on top of the mandibular condylar, it can create any of the previously mentioned symptoms, indicating TMD. The position of the disc on top of the condyle protects the bone from wear and tear. An injury to the disc, whether it is a tear to the posterior ligament that stabilizes the disc in place or a tear within the disc itself, can leave the mandibular condyle vulnerable to degenerative changes and can lead to arthritis.

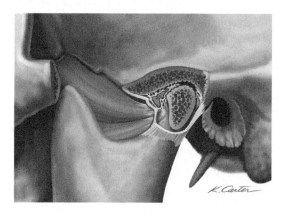

The above image shows the lateral pterygoid muscle attaching directly to the TMJ disc. If this muscle is overstretched secondary to whiplash of the mandible from a head injury or neck strain, a tear can occur in the ligaments stabilizing the disc. This image shows a complete tear above the mandibular condyle.

Without the protection of an intact and stable disc, bony changes of osteoarthritis on the condylar head of the mandible can occur creating instability in the joint.

Any trauma to the structures involved in breathing and swallowing also have a direct effect on the development of the face. For example, if there is a heavy blow to the abdominal area causing the patient to lose their breath, the thoracic diaphragm decreases its full capacity for exhalation/inhalation. Shallow breathing typically leads to open mouth breathing, which we all now know affects the development of the face and can create TMD.

Hypermobility syndromes can result in TMD. This syndrome affects the joints and bones, allowing them to go beyond the normal range. This disorder has also been named double-jointed or loose-boned. The syndromes are thought to be genetic but there is a commonly missed connection with dysbiosis (gut inflammation and malabsorption) that can also create weak ligaments. Nutrients delivered in the blood are prioritized to the organ and muscles. The connective tissues, including the ligaments, receive what is left over. If a person's gut is compromised with a decrease in absorption of nutrients, this creates a potential condition of weak ligaments. I commonly see gut inflammation associated with hyperflexibility in the patients I treat. As the mandible is suspended by ligaments and muscles, it has an increased risk for injuries in these hypermobility syndromes. We also see an increase in compensating muscle contraction with hypermobility, as the muscles over-function for the under-functioning weak, overstretched ligaments. Practitioners need to become educated in how to assess hypermobility syndromes and learn to treat underlying pathologies in order to be able to treat these patients' TMD symptoms.

Muscle tighten plays a role in TMJ disorders. I have found low magnesium and over-contracting of muscles a common cause and obstacle to heal TMD. As muscle fibers contract in a shortened condition the joint space is decreased and the "wear and tear" in the joint creates an increase in degenerative changes. A "chicken egg" experience is created as the presence of joint inflammation from over-contracted muscles creates ongoing muscle contractions as a protection mechanism for the joint. Just as our leg muscles would tighten up to protect from walking on an inflamed ankle joint. Jaw muscle tightness can also be the results of overall postural muscle tightness. When postural muscles tighten, the jaw muscles also tighten, especially the temporalis muscles, which are the primary postural muscles for the lower jawbone. Similarly, jaw muscle tightness can also be caused by an unstable bite. Without a stable occlusion to rest on and work against, the jaw muscles cannot function normally or relax fully. They undergo increased resting tension, because the muscles hold themselves constantly on guard as if they were applying continuous low level tension to stabilize the joint. I have found that intramuscular or intravenous injections of magnesium to be extremely helpful for my patients with globally tight muscles. It has been the "game changer" for many of my patients.

Anxiety, fear and sympathetic overload (i.e. stress!) can worsen any muscle-related conditions in the body but it has an especially powerful effect on TMJ disorders because of the imbalance in contraction capacity between jaw opening and jaw closing muscles. In other parts of the body, our joints rest between the balanced contracted muscles for the opening and closing of the joint. But, the TMJ muscles of closing are immensely more powerful and larger in their contraction capacity than are the opening muscles of the TMJ. Thus when there is an overall increase in body muscle contraction the closing TMJ muscles are that much more over-contracted than the opening muscles. This over-contractual balance is evident on physical exam as an increase in the antegonial notch on the mandible. It is also seen on an X-ray or CBCT scan indicating TMD.

The epidemiologic predilection of TMD in women is striking and worth mentioning. In the general population, TMD is two times more prevalent in women than in men, and in the patient populations TMD has a female-to-male preponderance as high as 10:1.[29] [30] [31] Also interestingly, unlike similar diseases in other joints, which have a greater female predilection but occur postmenopause, a large proportion of women with TMD is between eighteen and forty-five years of age.[32] [33] [24]

The above information about the importance of the functioning of the jaw joint and the temporal bone motion ties together the need for treatment of the joint and craniofacial cervical (whole body!) dysfunction in all patients with head injuries, whiplash injuries, neurodegenerative diseases, movement disorders and more. The TMJ is the accommodator for the changes in the cranium, cervical vertebra, vision, dental occlusion, tongue function, and neuromuscular integration, as well as vagus nerve function. Basically, it's a really important joint to learn how to assess and treat with an integrative collaborative approach. It connects the face with the cranial bones, hyoid and cervical vertebrae. What is obvious about this joint and commonly missed is it stabilizes the functioning and volume (space) of our airway as well as swallowing, chewing, speech and cervical stability. We need our jaw joints to have optimal functioning for optimal capacity for airway, chewing, swallowing and brain drain for optimal neurological functioning. So, it's important to learn how to assess and treat TMD with an integrated biocompatible approach.[35-43]

TMD, glymphatics (the brain drain), and neurodegenerative diseases

TMD, cranial somatic dysfunction, neurodegenerative diseases, and glymphatics – is there a connection?

In 2015, scientists discovered that the brain has a functional lymphatic system that runs alongside the venous system.[44] This was a huge discovery, as it was previously thought the brain did not have a lymphatic system. It sparked a re-appraisal of our approach to understanding and treating neurodegenerative diseases. It also provided a paradigm to understand the relationship between head injuries, cranial somatic dysfunction, TMD, ankyloglossia, malocclusions, torticollis, neurodegenerative diseases, and the brain drain. All of the above could be the consequence or the etiology of impeded cranium motion and glymphatic drainage. We are just beginning to understand the interface and relationships of all of the above pathologies, and thus perhaps move one step closer to creating holistic integral treatments for the cure.

The venous and lymphatic systems in the body depend on movement for drainage. Our blood is compartmentalized within a system of tubes (arteries) that are innervated by the nervous system to create the compression/decompression to stimulate fluid movement. The venous and lymphatic systems, in general, are not innervated by the nervous system, and the vast majority of the lymphatic system is not contained within vessels. They both rely on local pressure changes in the soft tissues to drive fluid drainage. Without these local pressure changes, lymphedema and venous congestion (i.e. swelling) can occur. This means that our bodies need to have pliability, elasticity, and ease of motion in our soft tissues (to be in a "Gumby" state, see Chapter 2, page 88) to allow for pressure changes to drive our lymphatic and venous drainage. When the tissues are hard and rigid, the elongation to shortening distance is limited and thus the local pressure change is minimal, with less fluid drive.

So, our lymphatic and venous systems have the greatest potential for motion for maximal compressive forces when our tissues are flexible and elastic. For example, the largest lymphatic vessel is just below the central tendon of the thoracic diaphragm, giving the area optimal compression/decompression and pumping movement with each breath. Lymphatic and venous systems typically lie between muscles, using the contractions of the muscles to act as a piston for the fluid drive. The glymphatic system, which drains the lymphatic systems out of the brain, does not lie between any muscles but instead runs alongside the venous system within fascia. The dura is the redundant thickened fascia that provides the "highway" for glymphatic and venous flow from the brain to exit the cranium. The cranial motion of the brain, dura, cerebrospinal fluid, and bones all provide a subtle motion that is thought to aid in the venous and glymphatic drainage. It is also postulated, at this time, that the heart contraction provides a pressure gradient to the venous/glymphatic fluid drive. Not only is the motion of the cranium important for effective fluid drive to move the toxins and by-products of cellular respiration out of the brain but the exit out of the cranium also needs to have a pliability of fascia for optimal drainage.

Most of the venous and glymphatic fluid drains out of the cranium through a space between two bones called the jugular foramen. Instead of using the compression/expansion motion of muscles as the initiation of the pressure changes for the fluid drive, here we see the body using the compression/expansion of the motion of the cranial bones, which is also augmented by a functional swallow. This fossa is occupied with fascia, the internal jugular vein, and cranial nerves 9, 10, and 11. As the cranium bones move with an expansion/contraction swelling motion of 0.29 microns to 1.5 millimeters,[45] [46] [47] the pressure change created in this fossa and fascia pumps the venous and lymphatic fluids, and aids in draining them out of the cranium into the deep cervical (neck) lymph nodes. Optimal brain drain is dependent on the motion of the cranial bones, dural membranes, and central nervous system for removing toxic waste products out of the brain. It makes sense that a hindrance to the motion in the craniofacial cervical complex can compromise optimal brain drain. Health is motion and motion is Life!

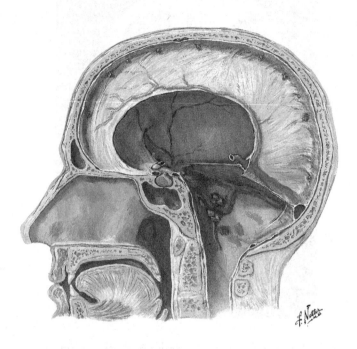

The above image shows the dural membrane that houses the venous and lymphatic system of the cranium. As the cranial bones move, the venous and lymphatic system receives pressure changes that provide some of the motion for the fluid drive draining the brain of its toxins.

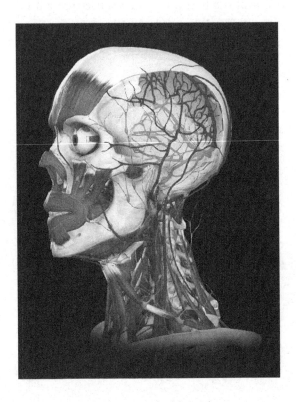

The above image shows the venous and lymphatic system in the cranium and neck. The glymphatic system runs alongside the venous system and follows the same drainage pattern. Not shown above is the membranous dural structures that envelop the venous and lymphatic fluids of the cranium. Both venous and lymphatic systems are dependent on motion for drainage. This motion is partially provided by the cranial rhythmic impulse, which includes movement of the cerebrospinal fluids, and the motion of the central nervous system, dura, and cranial bones (as well as the fluctuation of the sacrum).

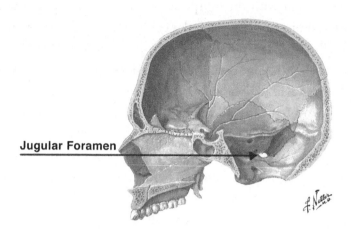

Jugular Foramen

The jugular foramen is a space between the occipital and temporal cranial bones. Most of the venous and lymphatic drainage of the brain exits the cranium through this space and drains into the deep cervical lymph nodes located behind the sternocleidomastoid muscle. Cranial nerves 9-11 also exit the cranium through this space.

If we add in the glymphatic piece of the puzzle, already knowing that the motion of the temporal and occipital bone plays a significant role in the brain drain...wow!...there is a potent, potential connection between TMD, ankyloglossia, myofunctional dysfunctions, malocclusions, torticollis, and neurodegenerative diseases. How do all these pathologies connect? They are all dysfunctions of the craniofacial cervical complex, and the causes of various pathologies. TMD, ankyloglossia, myofunctional dysfunctions, and malocclusions are all dysfunctions that affect each other. The interface of all these pathologies is tongue function. For example, an anterior tongue thrust is associated with TMD, ankyloglossia, and malocclusions. When the tongue moves forward during a swallow, the mandibular condyle follows in a forward translation motion with a deficient rotational movement. A normal movement of the mandible during opening is initially a rotation downwards of the mandibular condyle, then a translation forward. The diminished rotational component with the overpowering forward motion on opening creates a flattening of the mandibular condyle, as typically seen on X-ray and CBCT scans. The same tongue thrust occurs with ankyloglossia as the tongue's full range of motion is restricted; instead of an upwards and backwards contraction motion during a normal swallow, the tongue thrusts forward, creating TMD. Stated simply, atypical swallows and tongue thrusts are the most common etiologies of malocclusions. Narrow palates are created secondarily to a deficient tongue-to-palate resting position. A tooth position is created by the sum of all the vector forces, from the soft tissue muscle contractions of the face and tongue during swallowing, chewing, and at rest; as well as the position of the maxilla, mandible, and the craniocervical complex in relation to one another.

Now let's understand the connection between TMD, ankyloglossia, myofunctional dysfunctions, malocclusions, torticollis, and neurodegenerative diseases. A fulcrum of connection of these pathologies may be temporal bone motion and position. We have already discussed the importance of the temporal bone motion in relation to creating a pressure change in the fossa that contains the lymphatic drainage from the brain. So, it would be logical to conclude that problems that create temporal bone dysfunction will affect optimal glymphatic flow.

TMD involves a restriction of movement not only in the joint tissues (i.e. discs) but also the temporal bone motion itself. No matter what the cause of TMD, if the joint is compromised, the temporal bone will have some positional or movement dysfunction. Many of the muscles that open and close the mandible are attached to the temporal bone. Asymmetrical contraction of these muscles can change not only the position of the temporal bone within the craniofacial cervical complex but also change its motion capacity. Any condition that creates a decrease in joint space, with a compromise to mandibular and temporal bone motion, has the potential to affect optimal brain drain. As the lymphatic system is completely dependent on pressure changes in the local soft tissues created by movement in the musculoskeletal system, a dysfunctional movement of a bone will decrease the pressure needed to move fluid. TMD is the pathology of the joint that connects the temporal bone to the mandible. Compromise to either, logically results in less optimal brain drain.

Ankyloglossia is a restricted motion of the tongue. How does this condition affect temporal bone motion? The muscle which directly connects the tongue to the temporal bone is the styloglossus muscle, which is involved in contracting the posterior tongue to the soft palate. This action not only augments the cranial motion through compression of the sphenobasilar suture, but also rotates and stimulates the temporal bone's motion, creating a pressure change at the jugular foramen and a brain drain experience. The act of a functional swallow involves not only the tip of the tongue being in contact with the hard palate, but also the posterior tongue compressing into the soft palate, stimulating and augmenting the cranial motion and the glymphatic system. Here we have a connection between myofunctional dysfunctions (all dysfunctional swallows) and a lack of compression through the palate into the cranium. TMD can be created by an anterior or a lateral tongue thrust. The less optimal compressive forces to the palate decrease the cranial motion and most likely create a less optimal glymphatic flow.

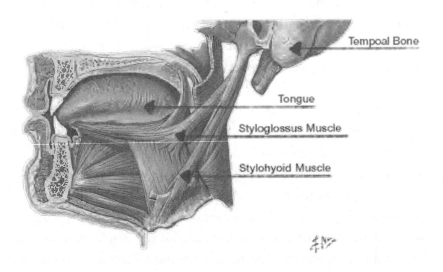

This picture shows the styloglossus muscle connecting the intrinsic muscles of the tongue to the temporal bone. Asymmetrical aberrant contraction of this muscle can create temporal bone malpositions and dysfunctional movements that in turn may affect the compressive forces within the jugular foramen (the space between the temporal and occipital bone), decreasing optimal venous and lymphatic drainage.

All malocclusions affect temporal bone motion and position, as well as other cranial bones, because the dental occlusion is the main horizontal stabilizing joint of the craniofacial cervical complex. The clearest example is a posterior or lateral crossbite where the maxillary teeth occlude inside the mandibular teeth. This occlusion literally locks the temporal bone into internal rotation with decreased excursions into internal and external rotations. An osteopath who has not been trained in dental osteopathy will not know to look for the dental occlusion as the cause of the temporal bone dysfunction and unfortunately for the patient, will continue to treat osteopathically without a cure. These patients need the ALF Approach of an ALF appliance, myofunctional therapy, and treatment from a trained ALF osteopathic physician.

There is clear evidence that patients who have experienced a traumatic brain injury (TBI) are more prone to neurodegenerative diseases.[48] [49] Head injuries are a risk factor for Alzheimer's.[50] The osteopathic perspective is that the movement of the central nervous system, the dural membranes, and the cranial bones have been restricted to their inherent motion through the compressive forces of an injury and thus brain drain or glymphatic flow has been compromised. When there are obstacles to brain drain, products from normal cellular respiration (i.e. growth or regeneration) become toxic waste products and build up within the brain, killing the surrounding healthy brain cells and leading to neurodegenerative diseases. Almost all neurodegenerative diseases are associated with the accumulation of these cellular waste products in the brain. The literature points out that a previous TBI may be one of the many antecedent events that contributes to the etiology of all of the neurodegenerative diseases including but not limited to Alzheimer's, ALS, and Parkinson's, to name a few.[51] There is reason to question whether the intra oral restrictive functions (ankyloglossia, tongue thrusts, myofunctional dysfunctions) are an underlying etiology for the limited neuroplasticity/ healing experienced by some of our patients with traumatic brain injuries.

A study was done on rats who had their deep cervical lymph nodes removed, which leads to cerebral edema.[52] This showed that an impediment or blockage to the outflow of the brain drain, which are the lymph nodes that lie in the deep cervical lymphatic chain, created a backup of lymphatic flow and thus led to cerebral edema. So, having an "open" outflow, which includes soft mobile cervical tissue, helps to keep the brain draining and healthy. There also needs to be freedom in movement in the front of the neck (scalenes and SCM) for optimal draining. The pliability of the sternocleidomastoid muscles is specifically very important for optimal brain drain because the deep cervical lymph nodes are located just underneath this muscle. If these muscles are over-contracted, inhibiting flexibility in the tissue, the lymphatic and venous drainage can be compromised with respect to their fluid drive and drainage. This is clinically significant when treating torticollis or forward head posture syndrome, as these conditions create an over-contraction of the cervical muscles and thus restrict lymphatic flow.

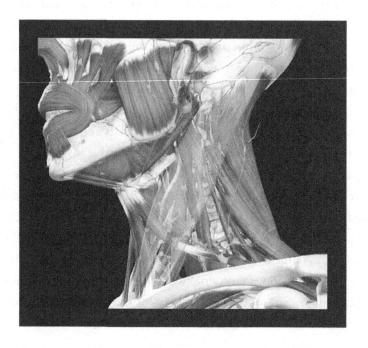

The above image shows the lymphatic system as nodes connected by vessels. The large diagonal sternocleidomastoid (SCM) muscle is faded to reveal the deep cervical lymph nodes underneath the muscle, which receive lymph drainage from the brain.

Interestingly, our glymphatic drainage happens almost exclusively during sleep.[53] When we are awake our glial cells (brain cells) expand, which reduces the space between the brain cells (extracellular matrix). While asleep, the glial cells contract, opening the spaces and increasing the flow of the cerebrospinal fluid (CSF). The extracellular space opens about 60% between sleep and wakeful times. Numerous compounds and waste products build up in the brain during waking hours including toxins like amyloid-beta, which is associated with Alzheimer's disease.[54]

Suboptimal sleep relates to suboptimal glymphatic drainage. Somatic dysfunction in the cranium will create a suboptimal discharge of toxins from our brain. The toxins build up in our brain, killing healthy neurons, and thus we have the connection between optimal craniofacial motion, the brain drain, and healthy neurons.

The new exciting horizon for the ALF Approach is treating patients with neurodegenerative disease from mild dementia to the more debilitating later stages of Parkinson's and Alzheimer's. As stated previously in this book, the ALF appliance augments, stimulates and unwinds cranial motion and strain patterns. Any effect on the motion of the cranial membranes and bones will have an effect on optimal brain drain and thus a potential decrease or increase in overall neuro functioning.

The above perspective of the relationship between head injuries, cranial somatic dysfunction, TMD, ankyloglossia, malocclusions, torticollis, neurodegenerative diseases, and the brain drain is based on anatomical and physiological connections. Research is needed in order to confirm the logical connections of the above pathologies, so I present the paradigm here in the hope that it will stimulate research to proceed.

How chewing increases memory and affects neurodegenerative disease

Risk factors for developing Alzheimer's disease include not only head injuries but also loss of tooth contact.[55] Many studies have investigated the occlusal-masticatory function (chewing) effects on brain function. In one study, molarless rats were given the task of finding their way through a maze.[56] It became apparent that loss of the mandibular vertical height in molarless rats was associated with decrease in learning, spatial memory, task performance, and dementia. Interestingly, these rats were shown to have less acetylcholine (ACh) in the hippocampus area of the brain. The hippocampus is part of the limbic system of the brain, which plays a role in the consolidation of information from short-term memory to long-term memory, and plays a role in spatial orientation. Alzheimer's disease also exhibits decreased ACh in the hippocampus. ACh is a neurotransmitter found in the gaps (synapses) between the neurons and is responsible for amplifying or inhibiting signals exchanged by the nerve cells. ACh also causes muscles to contract, activates pain responses, and regulates endocrine and REM sleep functions. Basically, it's important to not have low ACh levels in our brains.

Another study showed that impairment of spatial memory because of a decrease in ACh levels in the cerebral cortex was caused in 135-week old rats by tooth extraction.[57] A similar impairment of spatial memory has been reported to occur in aged mice by extracting or cutting the molar teeth at young ages, and also in adult rats by feeding them a soft diet after the weaning period.[58] [59] In these studies, both the neuronal density and synaptic formation in the hippocampus, the area of the brain that produces ACh, have been reported to decrease. One study looked at the connection between how tooth loss and a soft diet changes the cholinergic activity in the brain.[60] Again, the results of this study showed that the molarless rats (molar teeth were removed) showed a decrease of ACh in the hippocampus.

These molarless rats experienced a change in their dental occlusion, which created a clear change in their cognitive functioning. This is quite remarkable and should highlight that changes to the dental occlusion affect our health and functioning. We know that the dental occlusion helps maintain balance but here we find that molar tooth contact provides a sensory input to the brain connected to ACh productivity and the conversion of short term to long term memory. How the teeth make contact may stimulate the brain via the periodontal ligament through the trigeminal nerve and/or input from the TMJ. Removal of the molar contact changes the resting muscle length of the muscles of mastication, which are innervated by the trigeminal in an attempt to compensate for the loss of mandibular stability secondary to removal of the molars' contact. The position of the mandibular condyle shifts within the joint as a result of the shortened muscles of mastication, bringing the mandibular condyle into a more superior and posterior contracted position. It is unknown what exact sensory input is feeding into the brain with the change in occlusion, but we can be sure that it is the trigeminal nerve that is playing a main role.

The above studies clearly suggest that the deprivation of the oral sensory input caused by the decreased mechanical loading of the teeth causes a decrease in ACh production in the hippocampus. This also suggests that there is a close relationship between the masticatory function and learning and/or memory ability. Mastication helps to maintain cognitive functions in the hippocampus, a central nervous system region vital for spatial memory and learning. There are multiple neural circuits connecting the masticatory organs and the hippocampus. Both animal and human studies indicated that cognitive functioning is influenced by mastication. Masticatory dysfunction is associated with hippocampal impairments and hippocampus-dependent spatial memory deficits, especially in the elderly. Mastication is an effective behavior for maintaining hippocampus-dependent cognitive performance, which deteriorates with aging. Therefore, chewing may represent a useful approach in preserving and promoting the hippocampus-dependent cognitive function in older people. Mastication (chewing) is important not only for food intake, but also for preserving and promoting general health. Studies have clearly shown that chewing gum increases memory; so much for not chewing gum in classes!

The development of the mandible is directly related to the amount of muscle contraction used in chewing. A study looked at the development of the mandible in rats, some of which were fed a liquid diet and others food that needed to be masticated.[61] After four weeks, the height and width of the mandibular fossa and the width and length of the mandibular condyle were smaller in the rats on a liquid diet. The cartilage layer in these areas was also thinner at four weeks. The growth of the mandible is dependent on the masticating function. This is another example of how function creates the form. Chewing is needed to develop the mandible.

The "take home" message is to eat hard foods, chew well, and maintain a dental occlusion with a molar contact. This not only develops an optimal growth for the mandible, which is the most important bone for our airway, but also increases memory and cognitive functioning. One has to wonder what effect the increase in smoothies and soft infant diets are having on our developing children's faces, airway, and brain functions.

Connections between TMD, torticollis, and movement disorders

Spasmodic torticollis or cervical dystonia (CD) is characterized by sustained abnormal unilateral muscle contractions in the head and neck area resulting in abnormal positioning and posturing of the head. The cause is unknown and the condition is very painful. Traditional treatments are limited to Botox injections, and occasionally surgery is recommended. There may be a connection between TMD and spasmodic torticollis that involves the rotation of the upper cervical vertebra. Connections have been shown radiographically of patients with first and second vertebral subluxations (mal positions) have a malalignment of the TMJ. As the mandible rotates so do the upper cervical vertebra. Over 150 muscles and ligaments in the head and neck are used in the process of eating, and when the TMJs are malfunctioning (either through muscle pain or joint dysfunctions), the neck and shoulder muscles may go into painful spasm. This is one of the hypotheses given for the etiology of spastic torticollis.

The connection between torticollis and TMD lies in the attachment of the sternocleidomastoid (SCM) muscle to the mastoid process of the temporal bone. The muscles most commonly involved are the SCM, trapezius, and scalenes. As the SCM muscle contracts unilaterally it can displace the temporal bone into external rotation, which brings the mastoid process into a more inferior and posterior position, comparatively. This action also affects the upper cervical vertebra, creating malalignment of the spine and head position. The tongue tries to compensate for the overall body imbalance with an abnormal swallowing pattern or resting position. Because the mandible is attached to the temporal bone by the TMJ, it will move (rotate) to the side of the externally rotated temporal bone. This malalignment of the mandible can be assessed by looking at the upper and lower lip frenulums for alignment. If the upper and lower lips are pulled off the teeth, one will see tissue that attaches the lips to the maxilla and mandible. This redundancy of tissue is called a frenulum. Vertical alignment of the maxilla and mandibular frenulum is one way to assess the alignment of the mandible (see image below). To assess the position of the mastoid process, palpate the lowest point of the bone just behind the ears (mastoid process) on both sides and compare which one is lower (see image below). This will be the externally rotated temporal bone. Assessing the symmetry of motion of the mandible when opening and closing the jaw provides information on the position of the disc as well as the health of the ligaments and tendons of the TMJ.

When I treat patients with TMD I treat the entire body, with specific attention to the craniofacial cervical complex and pelvis. The healing of TMD cannot occur without integration of the entire soma. Even if a dysfunction is more prominent within one TMJ, the other TMJ is always incorporated into the treatment. A "right TMD" diagnosis does not exist. Both joints are affected in dysfunction as the bone functions as a single unit.

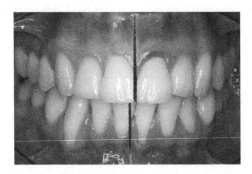

The alignment of the upper and lower maxillary frenulum can indicate a shift in the lower mandible, which is associated with TMD.

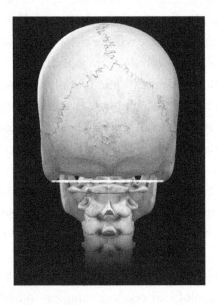

The above horizontal line indicates a leveling of the mastoid processes of the temporal bone. If there is an asymmetrical leveling of the temporal bones, the positions of the mandible in the temporal fossa will also be unlevel, resulting in the overloading of one joint leading to TMD.

A study reported cases of spasmodic torticollis that were treated with a dental appliance that increased the vertical height of the dental occlusion by using an appliance with acrylic pads on the lower teeth, creating more space in the TMJ and thus bringing the mandible into a more forward position.[62] Upon increasing the vertical dimension of the occlusion, there was a slowing and/or discontinuance of the symptoms of cervical dystonia. The proposed hypothesis for this reversal is that there may be neuritis of the auriculotemporal branch of the trigeminal nerve, which may activate the cells of the pontine region of the reticular formation (RF) in the brain, which is known for the control and deviation of head posture. The auriculotemporal nerve is positioned just behind the mandibular condyle. Research has shown that when the auriculotemporal nerve in the TMJ is stimulated, there is motor activity in the SCM and splenius muscles of the neck. This stimulus travels to the brainstem and activates the RF,[63] which can in turn cause the head and neck muscles to turn towards the same side as the stimulus. The etiology for spastic torticollis may be that these RF nerves are being constantly bombarded by noxious stimulus originating in the overstimulated nerves within the TMJ.

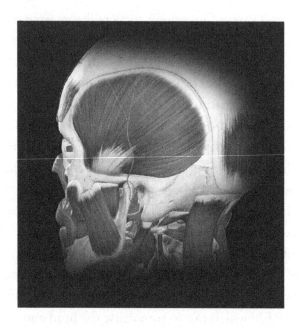

Note that the auriculotemporal nerve (a branch off cranial nerve 5) is in a vulnerable position behind the mandibular condyle. In conditions of TMD, the condyle commonly becomes displaced posteriorly and superiorly, potentially impinging on this nerve.

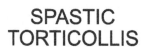

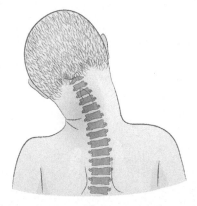

SPASTIC TORTICOLLIS

Spastic torticollis (cervical dystonia) is a disorder where the muscle of the neck contract unilaterally making the head turn towards the contracted side. The exact cause is "unknown" but the impingement of the auriculotemporal nerve secondary to TMD is a potential etiology.

If the mandible is pushed back with a retrotrusive orthodontics approach and/or is restrictive to forward growth and development secondary to restricted tongue function, the vulnerable auriculotemporal nerve behind the upper part of the mandible may become impinged, leading to an overactivation of impulses from the trigeminal nerve into the brain. This overactivation of neural input to the brain creates a "confused" or aberrant output response which may result in torticollis, an over-contraction of the cervical muscles. This overactivation of the trigeminal nerve may also be expressed as facial tics, grimaces and other aberrant muscle activations of the face and neck.

Examining the anatomical structures presented in the elderly population, one discovers that many have either had their posterior teeth extracted and/or have lost the youthful vertical dimension (maxillomandibular vertical interrelationship) that once existed through normal wearing and grinding of tooth structure.[64] This places the mandibular condyle into a more superior position within the glenoid fossa. It also displaces the condylar disk superiorly or posterosuperiorly, causing excess stimuli upon the retrodiscal tissues with its complex of blood vessels and nerves, particularly the auriculotemporal nerve fibers. Sensitization of the afferent input into the auriculotemporal nerve occurs. Impulses travel along the mandibular division of the trigeminal nerve and enter the spinal nucleus of cranial nerve 5. They stimulate the reticular formation (nucleus raphe and the medial reticular nuclei), which begins to initiate an inhibitory effect on the reticular formation, thus decreasing voluntary control of the cortex. Involuntary rhythmic tremors and imbalance of posture and gait disturbances can result.

As clearly stated in Chapter 9, a soft diet creates an underfunctioning oral masticatory system leading to an underdeveloped jaw. Not only does the mandible not reach its full growth potential but the height of the teeth is also diminished. That is, the teeth are actually shorter in height as the condylar part of the mandible is shorter, creating less space between the maxilla and mandible and thus less tooth height is needed to connect the maxilla and mandible to optimize chewing. Proportionally, the distance from the outermost point of the eye to the beginning of the ear should equal the distance between just under the nose to just under the chin (see image below) Most of the children I see in my practice are shorter from the measurement from under the nose to the chin. As this distance is smaller, the mandible is more compressed back into the joint space, which also affects the motion of the temporal bone. As explained above in the section of Glymphatics, the motion of the temporal bone is very important for the compression/decompression motion within the cranium to augment the drainage of the venous and lymphatic system of the brain.

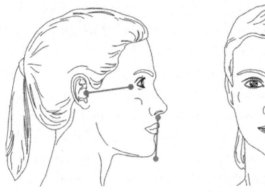 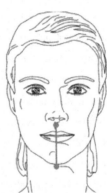

The above image shows a way to assess normal facial growth and development. The distance between the ear and the eye should equal the forward growth of the mandible. The point just under the nose to the tip of the lower jaw should equal the distance between the tip of the tragus (flap of tissue in the between the face and the "ear hole") and the outer part of the eye. This is an easy way to track your child's facial growth and development.

As mentioned earlier in this book, cranial nerves 9-11 exit the cranium between the temporal bone and the occiput. Any dysfunction in the motion of either of these bones can create an impingement syndrome for these cranial nerves. The accessory spinal nerve (11th cranial nerve) controls the motor function for the sternocleidomastoid muscle and the trapezius muscle, which are the culprits of over-contraction that create torticollis. This impingement can occur with birth injuries to the back of the head during the birth process (see Chapter 3). The common diagnosis associated with a compromise to cranial nerves 9-12 is called plagiocephaly. As many as 9 out of 10 infants with torticollis may also have plagiocephaly. This makes sense as plagiocephaly is simply an infant's head that is misshapen, usually secondary to birth compressive forces or molding to the mother's asymmetrical pelvis during pregnancy.

Here we see the connection between mandibular retrusion (backward position of the mandible), compression into the TMJ, activation of impingement of the auriculotemporal nerve or the 11th cranial nerve, resulting in spastic torticollis. As stated earlier in this chapter, the over-contraction of the SCM muscle could potentially limit the optimal drainage of the deep cervical lymph nodes that receive the waste toxins from the brain and create a potential back pressure with a tendency to increase cerebral pressure.

A number of electromyographic (EMG) studies have demonstrated evidence of the effects of the dental occlusion and the stimulation of the stomatognathic muscle function.[65] Basically, they were looking at how the teeth come together (dental occlusion) affects the muscles of swallowing, chewing, and facial expressions. The dental occlusal imbalances were shown to markedly alter EMG patterns, which indicate abnormal muscle contractions. Dental occlusal therapy can reduce the involuntary dyskinetic (abnormal muscle contractions) movements involving the face, mouth, and neck. There is a connection between malocclusion, facial tics, torticollis, and Tourette's syndrome.

As stated previously in this book, the dental occlusion plays a vital role in balance. Balance is defined as a state of equilibrium or parity characterized by cancellation of all forces by equal opposing factors.[66] This is the act of maintaining an upright posture (static balance) or in locomotion (dynamic balance or gait). This system depends on vestibular function, vision, and proprioception to maintain posture, to navigate in one's surroundings, to coordinate motion of body parts, to modulate fine motor control, and to initiate the vestibulo-oculomotor reflexes. These parts of the vestibular system provide our brains with information about changes in head movement with respect to the pull of gravity. Besides the visual, vestibular, and skeletal systems, which contribute to balance disorders, the dental (stomatognathic) system may also contribute to balance disorders. When all four of these systems are in coordination with one another, a person maintains equilibrium and balance, proper gait, and posture. It is recognized that there is a high association between the mandible, the neck, and body posture.[67] [68] The orientation of a patient's head and body posture (static balance) changes when the mandible is repositioned with a dental appliance, and it has also been determined that the dynamic balance or gait is also affected.

Stimulation of the TMJ tissues is known to evoke a reflexive response in the tongue and other craniofacial muscles.[69] It can also stimulate postural reflexes initiated through projections to the brainstem's reticular formation. There have been multiple studies concerning the maxillary-mandibular relationship and its positive or negative influence on a patient's posture when the proper vertical dimension is altered.[70] [71] [72] The significance of the findings in these studies makes it clear that there is an interrelationship between TMD, balance and gait disorders.

It is important for practitioners working with somatic dysfunction to clearly understand that malalignments do not necessarily indicate where the dysfunction originates. That is to say, if the right temporal bone is externally rotated compared to the left, the right temporal bone is not necessarily the "problem" side. The "problem" or dysfunction is determined by the area of the cranium that is exhibiting lack of motion. A structure's motion is the determining factor that defines the dysfunction as opposed to the position of a structure. This is a primary difference in philosophy between osteopathy and chiropractic. The osteopath is looking first for the motion of the structures as the chiropractor is assessing asymmetric position and treating it to alignment. The osteopath treats the dysfunction of motion, and restoring function and alignment is the consequence. The etiology of a misalignment is a restriction to motion. As motion and function is restored, the body is able to maintain its alignment without constant ongoing long term treatments. Reestablishing the motion or function addresses the underlying problems and avoids patients becoming "treatment dependent."

The TMD-vagus nerve-birth trauma and gut connections

Research is showing a potent relationship between gut and brain health! The neurophysiological connection for the brain-gut axis is through the vagus nerve. Given the compromised state of environmental collapse, it has become clear that we need to expand our diagnosis and treatment to include the microbiome and gut health. Soil and the human gut contain approximately the same number of active microorganisms. As biome diversity decreases in the soil, our guts also experience a decrease in diversity.[73] Food sensitivities continue to increase, with more people becoming gluten and dairy intolerant. Twenty four years ago when I first started my practice in medicine, it was rare to see a child with gut issues. Now, most children have some degree of inflammation (dysbiosis) and food sensitivities! It's essential for us to understand the gut-brain axis and learn how to diagnose and treat issues with it.

The vagus nerve is an essential part of the brain–gut axis and plays an important role in the modulation of inflammation, the maintenance of intestinal homeostasis, and the regulation of food intake, satiety, and energy homeostasis. The interaction between nutrition and the vagus nerve is well known, and vagal tone can even influence food intake and weight gain. The interaction between the gut and brain is based on a complex system that includes not only neural but also endocrine, immune, and humoral links. Interestingly, the brain–gut axis is becoming increasingly important as a therapeutic target for gastrointestinal and psychiatric disorders, such as inflammatory bowel disease (IBD),[74] depression,[75] and posttraumatic stress disorder (PTSD).[76] The gut is an important control center of the immune system, and the vagus nerve has immunomodulatory properties.[77] This means that the vagus nerve has a large influence on the immune system.

The vagus is a fundamental component of the parasympathetic branch of the autonomic nervous system. This nerve is largely responsible for regulating heart rate reduction, vasodilation/constriction of vessels, and glandular activity in the heart, lungs, and digestive tract; as well as control of gastrointestinal sensitivity, motility, and inflammation.[78] The vagus sends information about the state of the inner organs to the brain and thus affects the brain's output of instructions. There is preliminary evidence that gut bacteria has a beneficial effect on mood and anxiety, partly by affecting the activity of the vagus nerve. Because vagal tone correlates with a capacity to regulate stress responses and can be influenced by breathing, its increase through meditation and yoga likely contributes toward resilience and the mitigation of mood and anxiety symptoms.

Optimizing vagal tone is of utmost importance in our current condition of failing microbial biomes, increased GMO foods, nutrient-poor diet, and dysregulated autonomic nervous systems.[79]

Many studies cite the relationship between the vagus and the brain-gut connection. Both have an effect on one another. However, what has not been sufficiently acknowledged is the potential of vagal dysfunction from trauma, or impingement of the vagus nerve, resulting in the "vagal compression syndrome." As the vagus is the longest nerve in the body, it is most vulnerable to compression and thus dysregulation, which could produce a wide variety of symptoms, including vasovagal syncope, IBS, depression, and dysbiosis to name just a few. This connection is overwhelmingly missed because physicians and dentists are not asking the pertinent medical history questions to determine whether a head injury, birth trauma, cervical injury, or head forward posture has created cervical and temporomandibular dysfunctions. This syndrome is also widely overlooked secondary to our medical education over focus and fulcrum in pharmaceutical prescribing as opposed to neuromusculo-skeletal disorders requiring manual medicine as the primary treatment.

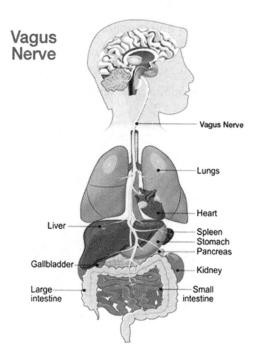

The above image expresses the vast influences the vagus has on organ and tissue functions.

The vagus has been named the King of the Nerves because of its vast domain of effects and influences. The vagus has also been called the "wanderer nerve" because of the long distance it travels from the cranium through the thorax into the abdomen. It is the longest cranial nerve, traveling between the neurocranium and the gut and is thus at greater risk for compressive forces and injury compared to the other eleven cranial nerves that travel shorter distances. The place of most common injury to the vagus is at the exit of the neurocranium at the jugular foramen, a space between the temporal and occipital bone; and the most common time of injury is at birth. Cranial nerves 9-11, along with the internal jugular vein and lymphatic vessels, leave the neurocranium through the jugular foramen. Interestingly, this foramen is simply a space between the temporal and occipital bone and contains fascial, vagus, glossopharyngeal and accessory nerves, and the internal jugular vein lymphatic vessels. The volume of this vital life supporting space is dependent on the position and motion of the occipital and temporal bones.

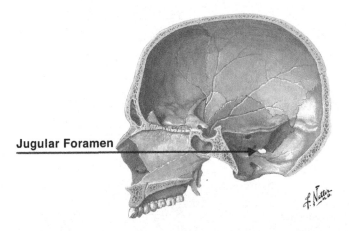

Jugular Foramen

The jugular foramen is a space between the temporal and occipital bones. This space is filled with fascia, nerves, arteries, venous, and lymphatic structures. Most of the lymphatic and venous drainage from the brain exits through this space and is dependent on cranial motion for optimal drainage. The glossopharyngeal, vagus, and accessory cranial nerves also exit the cranium through this space and are vulnerable to impingement secondary to cranial somatic dysfunctions.

Birth trauma, cervical whiplash injuries, head injuries, and TMDs (including all the etiologies of TMD) are the most common etiology to the compressive dysregulation of the vagus nerve that creates vagal compression syndrome. It is vital for practitioners, parents, and patients to understand the connection between birth trauma, whiplash injuries, head injuries, and TMD as a cause of vagal nerve impingement.

As explained previously in this book, compression of the occipital condyles at birth affects the hypoglossal nerve and concomitantly facial growth and development due to a weak and discoordinated tongue function (see Chapter 3). During the birth process, the baby's head compresses the mother's cervix in order to stimulate dilation and open the tissues. Any compromise to the opening of the cervix (secondary to malposition of the baby's head and other causes) that creates less stimulation to the tissues or lack of softening of the cervix can lead to an increase in compression into the baby's occipitoatlantal (OA) joint (the joint between the occiput and the first cervical vertebra) as the mother's unyielding tissue compresses the base of the baby's head. The occiput is the area of greatest compression at birth, as the sphenobasilar and condylar portion of the occipital bone articulates with the first cartilaginous joint between the cranium and the cervical vertebrae.

All other cranial bones at birth are "floating" in fascia and thus have no direct cartilaginous articulation. The OA joint is the first cartilaginous non-membranous connection between the cervical vertebra and the occiput (base of the head). It's the first joint that takes the majority of compression in a difficult birth. The OA joint involves three parts of the embryological portion of the occiput: the basiocciput and the two condylar portions of the occiput. These three embryological portions of the occiput, which are floating in fascia, articulate with the first cervical vertebra below to form the OA joint. The articulation of the OA on the first cervical vertebra is divided into two parts. The basioccipital portion holds one part of the OA articulation with the first cervical vertebra (atlas) and the condylar portion participates in the second part of the articulation with the atlas (see image below). The area of the OA joint is most vulnerable to birth compressive injuries secondary to its location as the first joint between the head and neck as well as the dynamic instability of the three (unfused) parts of the occiput, connected through fascia, creating one joint. The birth vector force through the top of the newborn's head into the occiput can create a multitude of compressive patterns through the displacement of any one of the three parts of the occiput. Any facial strain or displacement in one or all three of the parts of the occiput compromises not only the formation of the OA joint but also the competency of the hypoglossal canal that houses the hypoglossal nerve.

A birth in which Pitocin, vacuum extraction, or forceps are used, or that exceeds the "pushing stage" of two hours, is considered to be a traumatic birth from the baby's perspective. When an umbilical cord around the neck and/or a need for oxygen occurs at birth, it is considered a traumatic birth. If the occipital or temporal area of the baby's head is compressed, there is a potential for compression for the cranial nerves 9-12. The consequences of compression of these nerves include issues with swallowing, sucking, digestion and perhaps turning their heads (most common symptom is not being able to nurse on both breasts with ease), torticollis, spitting up after feedings, gas, and bloating. Basically, the colicky baby is the classic experience of the symptoms of occipital condylar compression. So, for every baby, child, and adult we see as a patient, it is imperative to ask the birth, nursing, and digesting questions to ascertain the functionalities of the cranial nerves 9-12 and assess whether occipital condylar compression was or is an influence on their health. (See Chapter 3 on birth trauma.)

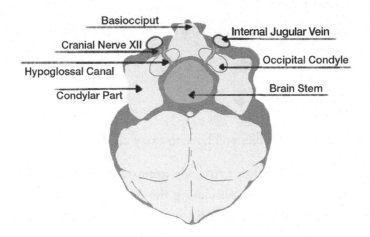

The above image shows an inferior view of the occiput with the occipital condyle (the circle with the cranial nerve XII passing through) separated between the condylar and basiocciput portions of the occipital bone. Compressive birth forces into the occiput can displace the unfused portions of the occiput and change the articulation of the first cervical vertebrae and occipital condyle, as well as create an impediment to the cranial nerve XII (hypoglossal nerve), which is the muscle coordination to the tongue. This will create a malocclusion.

Common symptoms of occipital condylar compression include:

- Nursing problems
- Difficulty sucking and latching
- Poor milk supply
- Painful nipples with nursing
- Baby falling asleep on the breast
- Reflux and vomiting
- Spitting up after nursing
- Colic
- Opisthotonus (arching of the head)

- Constipation

- Excessive gas (painful gas)

- Bloating

- Torticollis

- Difficulty staying asleep

- Irritability (babies you have to carry all the time!)

A detailed birth history is extremely important when assessing craniofacial development and considering the ALF Approach. This history is commonly missed by the dentist not trained in the ALF Approach.

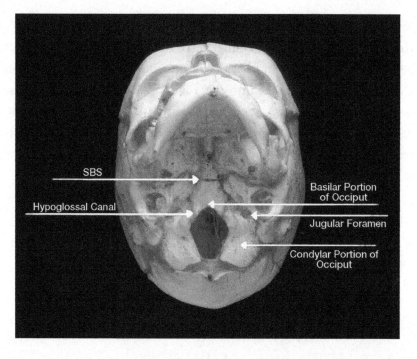

The newborn occipital bone exists in four separate parts at birth, as all the bones of the cranium are floating within the membranous matrix. The squamous, the two condylar, and the basilar portions of the occipital bone, are all connected to one another through the fascial system.

The two condylar and basilar portions of the occipital bone do not fuse together until after 8-9 years of age, and are still connected through the fascia between the separate bones at birth to stabilize the first cervical vertebra articulation. This is extremely significant, because any compression to the back of the head before 8-9 years of age could potentially create a significant fascial strain between the unfused condylar portions of the occipital bone, compressing cranial nerves 9-12 as well as compromising the glymphatic system.[80]

Any head injury, as well as cranial birth injury, to the base or side of the head that compromises the position or motion of the temporal or occipital bones can cause compression of the nerves, venous, and lymphatic structure passing through the space. A micro-fascial compression of a nerve creates dysregulation in its activation, leaving the nerve dysfunctional in its activation[81] and creating pathology. As mentioned in the section on glymphatics, any local tissue restriction to expansion and contraction will decrease the venous and lymphatic fluid flow, resulting in potential predispositions to neurodegenerative diseases.

As stated in the glymphatics section of this book, this is the area of greatest compression during a vaginal birth. Compression to the back of the head (occiput) may lead to a dysfunctional swallow (cranial nerve 9), dysfunction heart and gut innervation (cranial nerve 10), and torticollis (cranial nerve 11). The glossopharyngeal nerve helps to integrate a functional swallow. If there have been falls on the back of the head (compression to the occipital bone) or injuries to the side of the head (temporal bone area), there could be a twist in either bone, which could compromise the jugular foramen on one side of the cranium, thus compressing the nerves that exit the cranium.

It's not just the vagus nerve that could be compressed and compromised. Glossopharyngeal, vagus, and accessory nerves all transverse through the jugular foramen. The glossopharyngeal provides movement and sensory innervation to the palate for a functional swallow, and the accessory nerve is the activator for the sternocleidomastoid muscle and trapezius muscle. If these nerves are compromised the associated dysfunction is a disorganized swallow and torticollis, respectively. This highlights the connection to the syndrome of torticollis (wry neck), which can also be caused by a traumatic birth (from compression is the same area!).

It's interesting to note that a continuous over-contraction of the SCM, which attaches to the temporal bone, will position the temporal bone in a more internally rotated position, with the mastoid process more anterior and inferior, placing the glenoid fossa in a more lateral plane than the other temporal fossa. In order to maintain a balance to the vestibular and postural neuromuscular integrated system, the muscles of the mandible and cervical balancing system will have to compensate for the over-contracted SCM in order to maintain an upright posture stance. The overactive SCM can also compromise the motion of the temporal bone. This affects not only optimal glymphatic brain drain but also potentially compression of the other vital cranial nerves vessels entering and exiting the skull within the jugular foramen, which contains the vagus, glossopharyngeal, and accessory nerves.

The restriction to motion of the temporal bone can also affect the functioning of the inner ear as the three small "ear bones," also called ossicles, are housed within the temporal bone. Embryologically these three small bones (the smallest bones in the body) originate as part of the mandible but have separated out to give human beings a more refined hearing capacity. The stapedius and tensor tympani muscles create the tension between the ossicles, resulting in pressure changes that stimulate the action potential of nerves carrying information interpreted as sound to the brain. The stapedius muscle is innervated by the seventh cranial nerve and the tensor tympani is innervated by the fifth cranial nerve. Interestingly, both of these cranial nerves exit the cranium through openings called foramina within the temporal bone. As form and function are reciprocally related and interdependent on one another, one can appreciate the importance of motion of the temporal bone to support the function of the nerves passing through the bone.

An interesting clinical finding reported by Stanley Rosenberg, PhD, is that tension in the right sternocleidomastoid (SCM) muscle is associated with a deformation of the cranium described as a "flat back of the head."[82] This change in shape of the cranium is called plagiocephaly, which is a flattening in any part of the infant's skull created by prolonged pressure. This asymmetrical pressure could have been experienced in utero during growth, during the birthing process, or prolonged time on the baby's back misshaping the occiput (back of the baby's skull). Dr. Rosenberg found that in every client diagnosed with ADHD, or a diagnosis on the autism spectrum, the right SCM was tight and was associated with a flat occiput on the same side. Research published in the journal of Pediatrics reported that the plagiocephaly expressed as flattening at the back of the skull was present in a higher percentage of the children with autism and ADHD compared to normally functioning children.[83]

Another potential consequence of torticollis and overactivation of the SCM muscle is compression on the deep cervical lymph nodes, which are a chain of lymphatic tissue lying just beneath the SCM muscle. The majority of the lymphatics from the brain drain into these cervical lymph nodes, at least in rats.[84] Studies still need to be done to confirm that the glymphatic drainage is the same in humans as rats. A study done on rats where these deep cervical lymph nodes were removed resulting in cerebral edema points to the importance of having functioning deep cervical lymph nodes for brain health.[85] As mentioned earlier in this book, optimal lymphatic drainage is completely dependent on motion in the local tissue. So, if the SCM is overactive and contracted, there is less expansion/contraction elasticity of the muscle, which will affect optimal glymphatic flow and brain health. When an infant has torticollis and grows with this strain pattern, not only does it affect the development of the cranium, the TMJ, the dental occlusion, the vestibular ocular reflexes (to maintain upright posture), the alignment of the vertebra, the rotation of the pelvis, but even how we walk. It will also affect the capacity for the brain to heal from head injuries and detoxify itself at night from neurotoxins when they build up in the brain, creating cell death leading to neurodegenerative disease and dementia. So, let's make sure that we treat all babies with torticollis with cranial osteopathy.

The tongue also helps stabilize the TMD with thrusting activity. The myofunctional therapist attempting to rehabilitate the lateral or anterior thrust and swallow dysfunction efforts will be hindered if the underlying issue of treating the torticollis and temporal bone dysfunction is not diagnosed and treated first. A compromise to the accessory nerve is the etiology of torticollis. A detailed birth and trauma history will help to identify the patients who are at risk for occipital condylar compression. The obstacles are the overactive muscle contraction and temporal bone dysfunction. The tongue is moving to maximize joint stabilization in order to maintain optimal airway. This is another great example of the collaboration needed within the professions of dentistry, myofunctional therapists, and osteopathy. There is a connection between torticollis, TMD, and anterior/lateral tongue thrusts and these dysfunctions can affect vagal tone.

Neil Nathan, MD, an expert in Toxic Mold Sickness, and author of Toxic understands the utmost importance of an unimpeded optimally functioning vagal innervation in order for the mold toxic patient to detoxify adequately. A patient who has a history of head injury, whiplash injury, TMD, ankyloglossia, or torticollis may all be unable to tolerate the detoxification medication or treatments without an optimal functioning vagal tone. The basic osteopathic principle of "help the body help itself first" by removing obstacles of health before administering medications will optimize the patient's health to be able to tolerate medications or a detoxification process. I have treated many toxic mold patients with

TMD and vagal compression syndrome with the ALF Approach (in collaboration with an ALF dentist), osteopathy, and by administering platelet-rich plasma (PRP) to the TMJ for cellular regeneration and stabilization. When the vagus nerve is improving in its functions and is healing from the compressive temporal bone impact secondary to TMD, a detoxification process is less impeded. The osteopathic approach is to find and remove the obstacle to health so the patient is able to heal themselves. We approach our patients with the question, "How can I help you help yourself?" This osteopathic perspective is the paradigm of the ALF approach. First we create a functional neuro-cervical craniofacial complex and then we reassess what medicines or supplements are needed. We first optimize the individual's health by optimizing the physiological motion already inherent to growth, development, and health.

Another unrecognized area of potential injury is just in front (anterior) of the C1-C3 where the vagus nerve passes just anterior to the vertebra. Any cervical instability, hypermobility, or extended position of the first through third cervical vertebra could potentially compress the vagus nerve. There is only a 2-3 mm space between the anterior border of the cervical vertebra and the vagus nerve. Only a small dysfunctional forward motion is needed to possibly create vagal nerve compression syndrome, which could create a wide variety of symptoms including dysbiosis, vasovagal syncope, POTS, IBS, gastroparesis, mood swings, and mast cell activation to name a few!

Additional symptoms of vagal nerve compression include:

- Difficulty speaking or loss of voice
- A voice that is hoarse or wheezy
- Trouble drinking liquids
- Loss of the gag reflex
- Pain in the ear
- Unusual heart rate

- Abnormal blood pressure

- Decreased production of stomach acid

- Nausea or vomiting

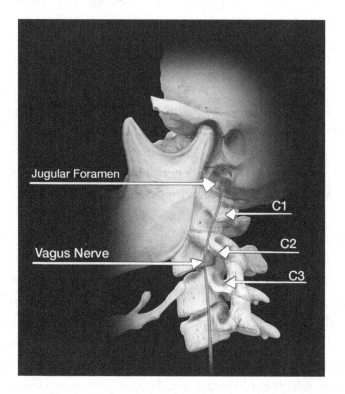

The vagus nerve exits the cranium through the jugular foramen and runs down the neck just in front of cervical vertebrae 1-3. A head forward posture could create an impingement of this nerve.

As the vagus is the longest nerve traveling from the cranium to the colon there are many areas of vulnerability to fascia strains affecting optimal function. The most common is, firstly, where the vagus passes through the jugular foramen into the neck region and secondly, in front of the upper cervical vertebrae where it can be affected by hypermobility and instability of these vertebrae. Two other common areas of compression are anterior cervical muscle over-contraction and thoracic diaphragm restriction. The vagus descends down the neck just behind the sternocleidomastoid muscle and in front of the three scalene muscles. If there is a head forward posturing, these anterior cervical muscles are over-contracted and could create an impediment on the vagus. The thoracic diaphragm is usually tight to extremely restricted with most of my patients. Our society seems to be over-driven in our sympathetic nervous system, resulting in short panting breaths which do not expand the thoracic diagram to its full extent, leaving the muscle in a state of chronically decreased range of motion. This large slip of muscle extends across the body, attaches to the lower six ribs and has ligamentous fascial attachments to every abdominal organ. If it is contracted, the opening within the diagram is more compressed so this can potentially impinge on the vagus as it passes through. Worth mentioning here is also the profound effect thoracic diagram restriction has on the lymphatic system. The largest lymphatic vessel resides just beneath the central tendon (fascia) of the thoracic diaphragm. Why? Because the lymphatic system is completely dependent on compression/decompressive forces to create a fluid drive for drainage. As most people are compromised in their breathing, the thoracic diaphragm is more restricted and thus there is a compromise to the lymphatic flow from behind the diagram into the thoracic cavity.

The polyvagal theory

The polyvagal theory is worth presenting as it provides an understanding of the vast influences associated with vagus function, also called "vagal tone." This theory emphasizes the importance of optimal vagal function, which can be compromised from a traumatic birth, a traumatic brain injury or head injury, TMD, or instability (hypomobility) of C1 and/or C2. The vagal tone can affect a person's overall emotional well-being and sense of safety.

The theory was introduced in 1994 by Dr. Stephen Porges, director of the Brain-Body Center at the University of Illinois at Chicago. According to the theory and its increasing evidence base, the autonomic nervous system is interconnected with and sensitive to influences from neuronal input from the body to the brain, called afferent influences.[86] The polyvagal theory claims that humans have physical reactions, such as cardiac and digestive changes, from the body's neural input. An example of the polyvagal theory is facial expressions changing cardiac and digestive functions.[87]

The vagus nerve serves the parasympathetic nervous system, which is the calming aspect of our nervous system. The parasympathetic part of the autonomic nervous system balances the sympathetic active flight, fight, and/or fright part, but in much more nuanced ways than was previously understood. Before polyvagal theory, our nervous system was pictured as a two-part antagonistic system, with more activation signaling less calming and more calming signaling less activation. Polyvagal theory identifies a third type of nervous system response that Porges calls the social engagement system, a mixture of activation and calming that operates out of a multitude of nerve influences. This social engagement system helps us navigate relationships and provides a foundation for the essential human experience of feeling connected and bonded.

Polyvagal theory explains that both branches of the vagus nerve calm the body, but in different ways. Shutdown, or freeze-or-faint, occurs via the dorsal branch of the vagus nerve. This reaction can create the sensation of fatigued muscles and lightheadedness. When the dorsal vagal nerve shuts down the body, people can experience immobility or a dissociation emotional state. In addition to affecting the heart and lungs, the dorsal branch affects body functioning below the diaphragm including digestive issues.

The ventral branch of the vagal nerve affects the body functioning above the diaphragm. This is the branch that serves the social engagement system. Also interestingly, the ventral vagal activity takes milliseconds, whereas the sympathetic activation takes seconds and involves various chemical reactions. In addition, once the fight-or-flight chemical reactions have begun, it can take our bodies 10–20 minutes to return to our pre-fight/pre-flight state. The ventral vagal nerve can make quicker adjustments between activation and calming.

Porges chose the name "social engagement system" because the ventral vagal nerve affects the middle ear, which filters out background noises to make it easier to hear the human voice. It also affects facial muscles and thus the ability to make communicative facial expressions. Finally, it affects the larynx and thus vocal tone and vocal patterning, helping humans create sounds that soothe one another. When we experience our environment as safe, we operate from our social engagement system. We can connect and feel a sense of belonging and bonding, which creates a womb of safety and protection. If the vagus nerve was compromised during, for example a birth injury, the neuro activation can signal the entire body from a visceral perspective that there is danger and even life-threatening danger. The body can become "wired" to continuously react as if there is impending danger secondary to the traumatized vagal nerves even though the actual environment is no longer dangerous.

Since publishing *The Polyvagal Theory: Neurophysiological Foundations of Emotions, Attachment, Communication and Self-Regulation* in 2011, Porges has studied the use of sound modulation to train middle-ear muscles. Clients with poor social engagement system functioning may have inner ear difficulties that make it hard for them to receive soothing from others' voices.

Peter Levine, a colleague of Porges, has studied the shutdown response through animal observations and bodywork with clients. In *Waking the Tiger: Healing Trauma*, he explains that emerging from shutdown requires a shudder or shake to discharge suspended fight-or-flight energy. When they can sense that they are safe, they can shift into their social engagement system.

When clients are more present in their bodies and better able to attend to momentary muscular tension, they can recover from a shutdown response. Body-awareness techniques that are part of cognitive behavior therapy (CBT) and dialectical behavior therapy (DBT) can help trauma move out of dissociative, shutdown responses by encouraging them to become more embodied. Osteopathic treatment to address the compressed and injured areas of the vagus as well as provide "safe space" to embody the present moment can also provide profound healing.

As described by Bessel van der Kolk, professor of psychiatry at the Boston University School of Medicine: "The Polyvagal Theory provided us with a more sophisticated understanding of the biology of safety and danger, one based on the subtle interplay between the visceral experiences of our own bodies and the voices and faces of the people around us. It explains why a kind face or a soothing tone of voice can dramatically alter the way we feel. It clarifies why knowing that we are seen and heard by the important people in our lives can make us feel calm and safe, and why being ignored or dismissed can precipitate rage reactions or mental collapse. It helped us understand why attuning with another person can shift us out of disorganized and fearful states. In short, Porges' theory makes us look beyond the effects of fight or flight and put social relationships front and center in our understanding of trauma. It also suggested new approaches to healing that focus on strengthening the body's system for regulating fear responses."[88]

An integrative approach to treating TMD

The TMJ is a uniquely structured joint between the temporal bone of the cranium and mandibular bone of the face. This joint connects the head to the face. The head is composed of 29 bones: 8 cranium bones, 14 facial bones, 6 auditory bones (ear bones), and the hyoid. One can visualize these bones as "floating" in soft connective tissue which creates the integrated craniofacial system. This elastic fluid complex of 29 bones that form the head and face has an expansion and contraction motion associated with the flow of cerebrospinal fluid (CSF) and movement of the central nervous system. Each bone has a very specific motion determined by the unique micro architecture surface of the suture. The bones interdigitate with one another, with certain bones sliding over other bones. Some of the cranial sutures are beveled externally and some internally, which determines which bones glide over each other. That is to say, the position and shape of the sutures between the cranial bones determines the influences on the specific movement of each craniofacial bone.

There are movable sutures with soft tissue interconnections between the scalp and the inner cranial meninges that surround the bones (allowing the bones to "float" in a soft tissue matrix) of the craniofacial system, for which movement is vital for optimal health. In this complex, the TMJ has by far the largest range of motion of any of the other cranial bones. The temporal bone motion and position is the most important cranial bone to begin to assess TMD. No one bone or muscle can stand alone as any etiologies of dysfunction in the body; the whole system is a complex dynamic movement of biotensegrity. However, as we are limited by words (sometimes), we have to start with a limiting statement to bring focus to a starting point. The temporal bone houses the joint and provides the connection to the muscles that connect the head with the face, hyoid, cervical, sternum, scapula, swallowing, and chewing muscles into a complex integrated biotensegrity structure that stabilizes not only the dental occlusion and tongue function but also our precious airway space! The TMJ holds the mandible in a position to create our optimal or suboptimal airway. Interestingly, our "airway" is simply a space surrounded by collapsible soft tissue that attach to the maxilla (as well as the palatine bones and pterygoid plates), mandible, and anterior cervical vertebra.

The integrity of the TMJ is essential for maintaining stability to the craniofacial complex. It's another whole integrated, complex, and dynamically moving system, which helps to sustain and create the health of our brain via the glymphatic system, as well as the functioning of breathing, swallowing, and chewing. When one cranial bone is restricted in motion, the dysfunction affects the entire system. It is vitally important to have a flexible cranium with the capacity for motion. When treating TMD, assessing the motion of the temporal bones is crucial.

Osteopathic physicians practicing neuromuscular medicine have to look to the entire neuroskeletal system to find the obstacle to health. But as Dr. A.T. Still, the Father of Osteopathy, says, "We start with the bones." The health of the joints are of paramount importance for the integrity of the entire structure. Our joints provide the attachments for muscles and ignite our motion (the nervous system also needs to be engaged) thus allowing movement. If a joint is compromised, the muscles overcompensate and are in a constant state of overactivation in an attempt to compensate for the joint dysfunction. A tight muscle that is overactive because its partner "the joint" is dysfunctional creates an overall tight and weak muscle. The ligaments and joints need to be intact (to be able to open and close without restriction or crepitus) in order to stabilize the bone position and optimize the connection between bone to bone. This allows the muscles to move the bones with ease and not be in the constant state of "over functioning." No amount of soft tissue massage, neuro integration, remodeling, or release can integrate and permanently change the length of the muscle when the muscle is attached to a compromised joint. Addressing the compromised joint needs to be a part of the holistic treatment. The muscle has more adaptability and elasticity to take the lead in compensation for a dysfunctional joint. The muscle is doing the best it can to overcompensate for the joint that is under-functioning. The muscles will continue to be overactive in an attempt to provide maximal motion for the body. Having said this, there is great value in addressing muscle dysfunction through optimal expansion and contraction of the muscles so as to not over-contract a joint, thus creat-ing joint dysfunction. It's another "chicken-egg" situation. The muscles and joints are one in function with an interdependent relationship. In general, orthopedic surgeons overfocus on the joints and the physical therapists overfocus on the muscles.

TMD is a classic example of a pathology that interfaces between the medical and dental professions. Because the complexes of the TMJ can require coloration, just as the ALF Approach requires, to treat TMD with a dentist trained in treating TMD, an osteopathic physician who is trained and skilled in working with the dental occlusion, and a dentist skilled in the area of craniofacial dysfunction is required. The dental profession typically uses appliances; usually a variation of a splint, which brings the mandible forward and thus increases the TMJ space. This action lengthens the temporalis, masseter, medial, and lateral ptery-goid muscles, as well as opening the joint space, thus decompressing the TMJ. As the splint is in place, the muscles functioning can create an opportunity for these muscles to remodel their position of insertion and maintain the mandible in a more anterior position. As the man-dible is held forward, more space is created in the TMJ, and the lower splint opening the TMJ space will sometimes allow the displaced disc (positioned either forward, backwards, or sideways) to be captured and all is well! Unfortunately, many times the splint therapy is only effec-tive when the splint is in place. Without the mechanically held splint, which holds the mandible forward, the patient's symptoms relapse. Why is this? There are several potential reasons for the relapse and instabil-ity of the position of the mandible with splint therapy, which creates a "splint dependent" condition for the patient.

Most dentists are unaware of the utmost importance of the movement of the temporal bone in treating TMD. This is no fault of theirs. Just as an osteopathic medical education is lacking the integration of the importance of the dental occlusion in the treatment of headaches, neck pain and TMD, a dental education is missing the education on the influences of the soft tissues on the dental occlusion. This is another major missing piece to resolving TMD. The temporal bone is the bone that holds the attachments of most of the muscles of mastication and is the attachment for the ligaments of disc placement. The movement of the temporal bone and cranial motion needs to be restored in order to integrate TMD and stabilize the joint. The somatic dysfunction (soft tissue influence) of the joint, including the cranium, needs to be released and go through an unwinding process to reset to a normal physiological motion of the cranium before the joint can be stabilized without a mechanical splint holding it in place. It's essential for all TMD patients to receive osteopathic treatments for the craniofacial complex. The osteopathic question begins with "how can I help my patient help themselves?" This is where the osteopathic approach begins. What are the obstacles to health and how can they be removed before an intervention is given? Trauma and repetitive injuries can be resolved with osteopathic treatments first and then we can support our patients with dental splint and regenerative medical interventions to stabilize the craniofacial complex.

Brendan Stacks, DDS, is a well-known TMD orthodontist who quotes in his lectures "height heals." His process of sometimes dramatically increasing the vertical height of the dental occlusion via an acrylic lower splint and an upper ALF appliance has produced what could be called miraculous results. Why? The combination of the upper ALF maxillary appliance has the capacity to restore the inherent motion of the temporal bone by acting as a biometric tongue and biotensegrity support for the craniofacial complex. The upper ALF appliance is a 24-hour myofunctional, osteopathic, and dental appliance. It has the capacity to address and unwind the cranial distortions that are often the underlying cause of TMD. The lower dental appliance provides the height (sometimes many millimeters and centimeters high) with acrylic, thus increasing the mandibular vertical height, bringing the mandible forward. This decompresses the compression between the temporal and mandible and increases the joint space. This process alone can create tremendous relief of TMD symptoms because the compression on the disc is relieved rapidly.

However, the problem remains of how to rehabilitate the compromised ligamentous structure of the joint. With severe or even moderately severe TMD, torn or compromised ligaments that stabilize the disc on top of the mandibular condyle during opening and closing of the jaw can be present. All TMD cases have a compromise to some extent to the soft tissue of the joint. Some discs are able to be "recaptured" (the disc moves back into its position on top of the mandibular condyle) with splint therapy, the symptoms of TMD resolve and there is the restored ease of motion without pain, popping, clicking, or deviation of the mandible during opening and closing. Unfortunately, many of our patients are too compromised and their symptoms with dysfunctional motion remain with just splinting. I have found prolotherapy and platelet-rich plasma (PRP), which are injections made of dextrose (sugar) and platelet (the patient's blood is drawn and centrifuged to collect the platelets which are injected into the TMJ) used in the field of cellular medicine to be invaluable and the key to stimulate regeneration of the intra articular ligaments to stabilize the joint. Almost all of my patients that I have used PRP and the ALF Approach with for TMD have resolved their symptoms without a lifetime need for a lower splint.

To make matters more complicated, patients wearing lower mandibular splints for more than several months often develop bilateral (both sides), posterior (back teeth) open bites. This is when the molars don't occlude (touch together). A posterior open bite destabilizes the stability of the dental occlusion and requires more work from the muscles of mastication to organize and move the jaw joint, thus creating TMD. So, yes, the therapy most commonly used by a TMD dentist has the potential to create an occlusion that will continue to compromise the function of the TMJ by creating an open bite. Once the patient has a posterior open bite most dentists will use braces in an attempt to bring the molars back together. Now we are back with retrusive (backwards) traditional braces solving a problem that was created by a solution for the problem.

There is a "chicken-egg" experience between the temporal bone and mandibular condyle. If TMD is a result of injury and the patient has been treated soon enough, the osteopathic physician can restore normal physiological motion to the temporal bone and restore a displaced disc. If the patient continues, for months or years, with a dislocated disc with dysfunctional movement in the joint, the dental occlusion will shift and "lock in" the dysfunction in the jaw. The compensated occlusion will continue to create abnormal wear and tear in the joint as the condyle has not resumed its physiological position. The muscle of mastication will have to work overtime to stabilize what the joint is not able to stabilize. It is of paramount importance for the dentist to refer to an osteopathic physician who has been trained to treat the soft tissue influences of the mandibular complex before the teeth are moved to "alignment" without addressing the dysfunction in the joint. This situation has the potential to "lock in" the joint dysfunction into a dental chewing situation that could continue to aggravate and exacerbate the dysfunctional position of the mandibular condyle. Our body's joints create stability and our muscles move the bones. Intra-articular health is of extreme importance in order to allow the muscle to function optimally and not over-contract, causing the pain of TMD.

The dentist's perception is to change the occlusion in order to provide stability to the TMJ. This is no doubt very important but we also need to be aware that the joint itself needs to be rehabilitated with prolotherapy/ PRP or cold laser therapy to regenerate the traumatized ligamentous structures. It's another "chicken-egg" situation in this complex system called the human body. The TMJ needs to have a disc in place with healthy supportive ligaments holding the dynamic position of the disc, the dental occlusion needs to have a solid first bicuspid/molar contact to support the joint, and the muscles of mastication need to have symmetrical flexible contraction to move the mandible. All of these processes lead to either a functional growth or dysfunctional growth pattern for the mandible. The patient is not finished with the ALF Approach treatment if the jaw still has asymmetrical motion, pain with opening and closing, or any popping and clicking with opening/closing.

It is essential for the myofunctional therapist to be educated in assessing TMD. The tongue will not rest and cannot be "tamed" when there is a dysfunctional jaw joint present. One of the many responsibilities of the tongue is to stabilize the airway, which means stabilizing the jaw joint. If there are pops, clicks, pain, or deviations in the lower jaw when opening or closing, the tongue will apply pressure on the teeth (laterally thrust) to stabilize the joint. The tongue will not be able to resume its neutral position in the upper palate without a healthy TMJ. It's another "chicken-egg" situation with the structure function experience, with myofunctional dysfunctions creating TMD and TMD creating myofunctional dysfunctions. Both have to be addressed directly for the health of the whole system. A healthy mouth is a healthy body!

Cold laser therapy

I have used cold laser therapy since the early 2000s in my practice for many conditions including TMD pain, crepitus and recapturing the disc, by increasing blood supply to the injured ligamentous structures and decreasing the overactive compensating muscles.[89] The muscles of mastication are overactive as they are trying to stabilize a compromised joint. Splint therapy does not heal the compromised integrity of the joint, and the muscles are doing their job of contracting to compensate for an unstable joint. The perspective is to help the joint heal and regain its stability, thus allowing the TMJ muscles to elongate and strengthen to support the joint as a whole functioning unit.

The cold laser I have found most effective emits three wavelengths of red, infrared, and violet. More information can be found on my website www.drtashaturzo.com.

For two decades, I have treated patients with severe TMD. Some patients were cured and some were "stuck" in a dental splint-dependent TMD syndrome. These patient's symptoms were only resolved when they were wearing their splints. If the splint was removed, the patient decompensated with their symptoms of TMD. As I was experimenting with a variety of modalities to help our "splint dependent" patients in the late 1990s, I realized that the integrity of the soft tissue and disc of the joint was a pivotal missing component to stabilizing the patient and helping the tissues regain strength in order to stabilize the mandible in the new anterior functioning position. The muscle lengths and insertion sites had changed but the damage to the posterior ligament (which stabilizes the disc) and potentially other ligaments and tendons (including the attachment of the lateral pterygoid muscle onto the disc itself) were compromised. Even though there had been a change in the attachment of the muscles of mastication, the joint was not functioning as a healthy integrated stabilizing force for "airway" and chewing.

I needed to find a direct treatment to rehabilitate the joint and disc dysfunction. Dr. Nordstrom and I began injecting the TMJ with a variety of substances with prolotherapy and we gratefully began to see changes of increased stability of the joint. Many of our patients were able to throw away their lower splints! Over the years I have found the application of regenerative medicine with the injection of PRP to be one of the key missing pieces in treating TMD. To date, all of my TMD patients have improved using the collaborative combination of a craniofacial supportive dental appliance (the ALF), osteopathic treatments, cold laser therapy, and PRP.

CHAPTER 7

Food and the Face

by Traci Zimmerman Jones, DO

During my 8th grade home economics class, we did an experiment to begin our unit on cooking and nutrition. We had two cages, each with a pair of baby mice. We fed one pair fresh water and a mixture of mouse food containing seeds and fresh vegetables while the second pair's diet consisted of Kool-Aid and Fruit Loops. We observed what happened. The first pair of mice had bright eyes and shiny fur. They grew bigger and ran around their cage while the second pair of mice had sunken eyes, and dull, thin fur. They weren't as big as the other mice and they didn't run all around the cage. This was obvious after only a few days. My teacher stopped the experiment because the point had been made. We fed both pairs of mice fresh water and the seed and vegetable mixture. The second pair of mice began to grow and run around their cage. Their fur became thick and shiny and their eyes were no longer sunken. After a few weeks, there was no difference between the two pairs of mice. Through this experiment I saw firsthand the direct impact food has on health.

As a young person, I found all the conflicting information I saw on nutrition in the media confusing. One day eggs are bad for us, the next day they are good. One day fat is bad, the next day it is good. How does one sort through all of this information and decide what is the truth? I discovered the answer to this question when I read a book by Dr. Weston Price called Nutrition and Physical Degeneration. In this book, Dr. Price shows how the food we eat can positively or negatively impact our health as well as that of future generations. Let's take a closer look at his research.

Dr. Weston Price was a dentist who traveled the world in the 1930s to discover the secrets of healthy people. He studied the diets of people in 14 countries with very different climates. The diets of these people consisted of different foods depending on what was locally available to them. Despite the differences in diet, Dr. Price found people would remain healthy when they consumed their native diet, that is, whatever local food was available to them, foods their ancestors had eaten for generations. These healthy people had strong bodies and good facial bone structure with space for all teeth including wisdom teeth. They did not need braces. They had no cavities, yet they didn't brush their teeth, floss, drink water with fluoride in it, or have their teeth cleaned by a dentist. A strong immune system protected them from infections and chronic disease. They conceived, delivered and breastfed their children with ease and those children were healthy. They did not suffer from cancer, heart disease, arthritis, diabetes, mental illness or other chronic, degenerative diseases so common in our world today. The Native Americans didn't even have a word for "depression" in their language.

Below are Dr. Price's photos of healthy people. Notice the broad, u-shaped dental arches. This structure provides stability and balance not only for the mouth but also for the entire body. See how there is enough space for the tongue to rest in the roof of the mouth? When the tongue is in the roof of the mouth, a human being will breathe through the nose. This is the way we were created to breathe as you have seen throughout this book.

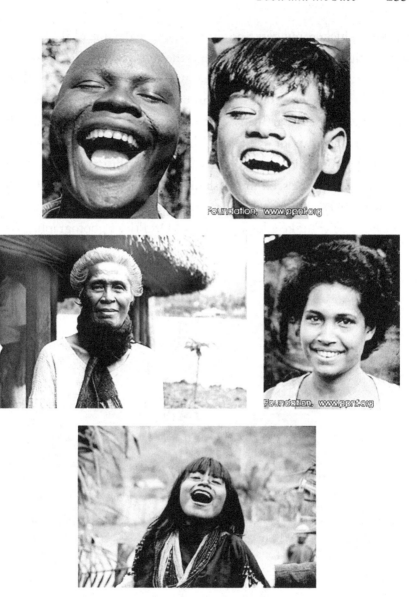

In addition to healthy people, Dr. Price also studied cultures eating refined and processed foods. Processed foods are those made from flour, sugar, and vegetable oils. Anything in a box, can or bag with multiple ingredients is a processed food. This includes cereals, donuts, pizza, crackers, chicken nuggets and even "homemade" bread if made with store-bought flour. When people ate these foods, Dr. Price saw them develop cavities and crowded teeth, as well as illnesses such as the flu and tuberculosis. They got sick with chronic and degenerative diseases like cancer, heart disease, arthritis, diabetes, and depression. Their children had birth defects, poor overall health, increased susceptibility to infections and chronic disease and suffered with infertility. The most striking differences could be seen in the shape of the faces. These children had narrowed faces and dental arches leading to crowded teeth. They also got cavities. Let's take a look at some of Dr. Price's photographs.

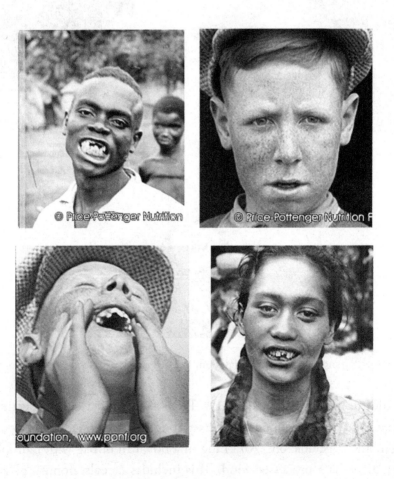

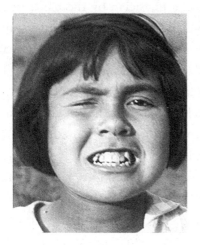 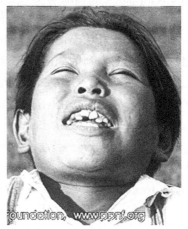

Now compare the broad dental arches from the photos of healthy people to the narrow dental arches of these people eating processed food. These people do not have enough space for all of their teeth and the teeth are in poor condition. The tongue will not fit in the roof of the mouth so instead it rests on the floor of the mouth. The lower jaw will tend to fall open and mouth breathing will occur. A mouth breathing child's jaws will not grow as big as they need to be and the child will grow up to have crooked teeth.

As we have seen in the photos above, good facial structure leads to good health and poor facial structure leads to poor health because facial structure influences facial functions vital to life such as breathing, drinking and eating. When the face is narrow, the openings to the sinuses will be too narrow for proper flow of air from the nose into the sinuses. This results in allergies, sinus problems and mouth breathing. There may be problems with the teeth such as cavities and the patient may have trouble swallowing if the tongue is not able to stretch enough to move into the roof of the mouth. This trouble swallowing can be a cause of acid reflux, yet patients suffering from this condition rarely realize how they swallow is the root cause of their problem.

In the same time frame as Dr. Price, a physician by the name of Dr. Francis Pottenger, Junior also conducted a 10-year experiment in nutrition. In his work, Dr. Pottenger raised cats, fed them different diets and made observations of their health. His findings paralleled those of Dr. Price. He discovered when cats were fed nutritious diets of raw meat and raw milk, they were healthy and their kittens were healthy and strong. When cats were fed poor diets of cooked meat and pasteurized milk, they developed degenerative diseases. In the wild, cats catch their prey and eat it raw. Their digestive systems were made to digest raw meat. The raw food diet Dr. Pottenger fed his healthy cats mimicked a cat's native diet. Dr. Pottenger also saw the same change in facial structure. Cats fed nutritious diets had big, broad faces while the cats fed poor diets had smaller, thinner facial bones. In this photo, the cat in the middle is from a cooked food litter and the cat on the right from a raw food litter. Notice the smaller face in the middle cat.

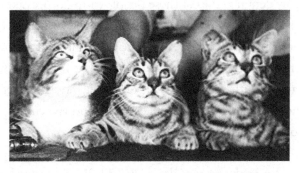

© Price-Pottenger Nutrition Foundation, Inc. All rights reserved. www.ppnf.org

The kittens born to the third generation of cats fed poor diets died shortly after birth. These animals could no longer reproduce.[1]

In another experiment, Dr. Pottenger took kittens whose parents had been fed poor diets and fed the kittens nutritious diets. He continued to feed the animals the nutritious diets and in four generations, the facial structures of the cats mirrored those of the healthy cats who had always been fed nutritious foods. Four generations of eating healthy food and the genes returned to normal! Read that sentence again. Let it sink in. Why is this so important? It illustrates the power of epigenetics. Epigenetics means "above the genes." This means different genes may be expressed depending on the environment. Just because you have the gene for a certain disease does not mean that you will definitely get that disease. For example, maybe everyone in your family has diabetes and you are worried you will get it too. Epigenetics shows us it is possible you will not develop diabetes. Genes can be turned on or turned off. In a healthy environment, the disease gene will not turn on and you will not get the disease. Through epigenetics, there is hope human beings can once again enjoy excellent health like the people Dr. Price studied.

After reading *Nutrition and Physical Degeneration*, my goal became to not just help my patients with their acute problems but guide them to achieve exceptional health. I taught them how to eat fresh, whole foods instead of processed foods. The results were impressive and, in some cases, medical problems present for 25 years vanished in a few weeks. Yet, I couldn't change the structure of their mouths. Someday, I thought to myself, maybe our facial structures will revert to the way they were meant to be. Would it take four generations as it had in Dr. Pottenger's cats? Would people be this patient? Would they really make significant lifestyle changes that would benefit their great-great-great-grandchildren?

Then I learned about the ALF, an amazing appliance that could change the shape of the mouth in the current generation to make it look and function like the mouths of Dr. Price's healthy people! This was the missing piece necessary to help my patients achieve the level of health I so desperately desired for them, the health that is critical for survival of the human race. We have now been eating processed food for four generations (since the early part of the 20th century) and rates of chronic disease and infertility are increasing. Are we on the way to ending up like Dr. Pottenger's poor-diet-fed cats who could no longer reproduce?

To understand the impact of nutrition on the growth of the human mouth, let's explore how it develops. Embryology is the branch of biology which studies the prenatal development of a baby from the moment egg and sperm join. Once an egg is fertilized, the cells begin to divide forming a zygote. The zygote becomes an embryo in the second week after fertilization and then all the organs begin to form. This process is complete by the eighth week after fertilization and then the baby is called a fetus. The structures of the mouth including the jaws, lips, and tongue form between the third and sixth week of pregnancy. This means that her baby's mouth has already begun to form before a woman even realizes she is pregnant! The primary teeth form in the 9th week, the beginnings of the permanent teeth in the fourth month, and the enamel on the teeth in the fifth month of pregnancy, long before they will be visible in the mouth.

In addition to his studies with cats, Dr. Pottenger also researched the impact of nutrition on the development of the human face. His studies showed poor diet in the first trimester of pregnancy can result in small teeth and inadequate development of the jaws. In this x-ray, the baby's lower jaw is too far forward and the middle of the face is underdeveloped. If untreated, this child will develop an underbite which is where the lower teeth come in front of the upper teeth when the person smiles.

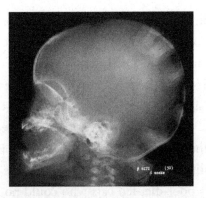

In this x-ray the baby's lower jaw is set back too far which takes up space for the airway and puts the child at risk for sleep apnea.

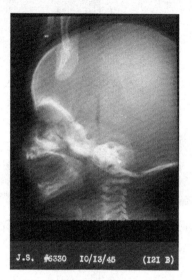

J.S. #6330 10/13/45   (I21 B)

Dr. Pottenger correlated these findings to a nutritional deficiency in the 7th week of pregnancy. He concluded the mother's diet is very important for the development of the face. Dr. Pottenger discovered children could show remarkable improvement in facial structure when following a nutritious diet while also encouraged to use their facial structures by chewing tough objects and making faces. Note the improvement in this girl from age 5 to 10 years.

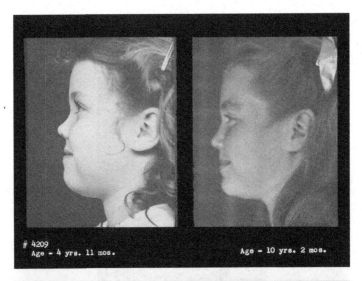

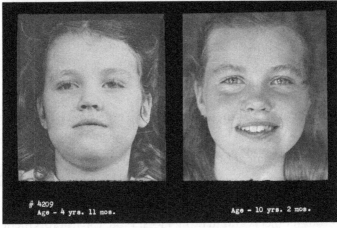

As osteopathic physicians, we use the term craniofacial structure to refer to the structure of the head (cranium) and face. Since craniofacial structure develops early in the first trimester of pregnancy, nutrient density of the mother's diet is important before she becomes pregnant because many nutrients are required to build the baby's body including facial bones. The father's diet is also important to adequately nourish the sperm before fertilization. Weston Price found all healthy cultures had special nutrition programs for their young people to follow in the

6 months before they were to be married and begin bearing children. These programs not only included foods rich in vitamins and minerals but also education for young people about why they should consume such foods. In this way, this information vital to creating health was passed down through the generations. In some cases, Dr. Price brought samples of these special foods back to his laboratory and analyzed them to demonstrate their exceptional nutritional value. For example, he found fish eggs eaten by girls and women of reproductive age in both Peru and Alaska to be a very rich source of vitamins and minerals. He also noted nursing mothers in Peru and Africa ate quinoa because it is rich in minerals and increased milk production.

While we may not have access to fish eggs today (nor want to eat them), we can still model our diet after the basic premise Dr. Price found to be true which is food in its most unprocessed state nourishes our bodies most effectively. The foods people ate varied depending on where they lived. For instance, Eskimos ate a lot of fish while African tribes ate plants from swamps and marshes. The diets of these healthy people did have some things in common. They consisted of a variety of fresh, whole foods grown in soil rich in minerals such as fruits, land and sea vegetables, nuts and seeds. Sources of animal protein included mammals, birds, reptiles, fish, crustaceans, mollusks and insects. Fat soluble vitamins (vitamins A, D, E and K) which are important for bone growth were obtained from butter, sea foods, cod liver oil, animal meat and organs and plant seeds. These foods also contain large quantities of essential omega-3 fatty acids which play a vital role in the function of many body processes including the cell membrane. All foods consumed were very nutritious containing all the vitamins, minerals and enzymes essential for human beings. Eating a wide variety of fresh, whole, unprocessed foods ensures we consume not only adequate amounts of macronutrients (protein, fat, carbohydrates) but also adequate micronutrients (vitamins, minerals, enzymes), essential both for general health and development of the face.

Thus far we have seen how the food we eat impacts the development of the face. The studies of Doctors Price and Pottenger demonstrate the importance of both nutritional quality of the food and how it is eaten. This starts preconception and is important throughout the entire lifespan. Just like we exercise our arms and legs we must also exercise our facial muscles. Babies exercise their facial muscles by nursing at their mother's breast while children and adults get this exercise by chewing and swallowing their food. Foods that we must chew more thoroughly, like fresh vegetables and meats, provide more exercise for our facial muscles than processed foods which tend to be softer and don't require much chewing. This is another way fresh, whole, unprocessed foods contribute to adequate jaw and facial growth. While fruit and vegetable smoothies and freshly made juices contain large amounts of vitamins and minerals, they do not exercise our chewing muscles. They can be part of a healthy diet, as long as we also include other foods that must be chewed.

Dr. Price observed different people eat different foods and yet remain healthy. How can we explain this and how can we use this information to determine what diet is right to bring each person living in today's world the same level of health of the people Dr. Price observed? To answer this question, we must look at how food impacts the body's biochemistry and physiology.

Osteopathic medical students spend many hours studying the autonomic nervous system. The autonomic nervous system controls all body functions that happen automatically without us thinking about it such as how fast or slow our heart beats and how we digest our food. There are two parts of the autonomic nervous system, sympathetic and parasympathetic. The sympathetic nervous system is our "fight or flight" response while parasympathetic controls "rest and digest" functions. These systems must be in perfect balance for our bodies to be able to find and maintain health. In this book you have learned about the osteopathic principles. The second osteopathic principle, that the body can heal itself, applies when the autonomic nervous system is balanced. Because the autonomic nervous system controls so many things that take place in our bodies, balancing it has a positive impact on many symptoms that seem unrelated.

Osteopathic treatment balances the autonomic nervous system, and so can food as demonstrated by Dr. Price. The healthy people he studied knew exactly what combinations of foods they needed to eat to keep their bodies healthy. When Dr. Price performed blood tests, the numbers confirmed an autonomic nervous system in perfect balance. These people had the fewest cavities in the teeth. The blood test results of those eating processed foods were not perfectly balanced. These people had more cavities.

Eating processed food unbalances the autonomic nervous system. One of the ways it does this is by its impact on breathing. Processed food creates more carbon dioxide which increases breathing and the more we increase breathing, the more likely mouth breathing is to occur.[2] Dr. Price observed Scottish children switch from nasal breathing to mouth breathing when their diets changed from their native oatcakes and fish to white bread and jam.

Dr. Melvin Page, a dentist, studied Dr. Price's work and applied the principles in his own practice in the 1950s. While his patients were hospitalized, he checked the levels of calcium and phosphorus in their blood after they had eaten certain foods. He found people would recover from disease when the calcium level in their blood was 10 and phosphorus level 4 for a ratio of 2.5. At this point, the body's minerals, autonomic nervous system, as well as hormones were balanced resulting in good health. Dr. Page studied the effect of various sweeteners on this balance. He found raw honey had the least impact while one teaspoon of regular white table sugar unbalanced the calcium phosphorus ratio for 72 hours! One can of Coke contains 9.75 teaspoons of sugar so a person consuming just one can of Coke daily will never have balance in his or her body. It is not only sugar but all carbohydrates that affect the body's mineral-autonomic nervous system-hormone balance. This is the second way the standard American diet (SAD) filled with simple carbohydrates from sugar and flour destroys health, by unbalancing the autonomic nervous system. Dr. Page's food plan consisted of unlimited servings of vegetables, especially leafy green vegetables like lettuce, spinach and kale. It also included protein from meat, poultry and fish, as well as limited servings of nuts, seeds and fruit. Grains were not included in the food plan due to their high carbohydrate content. Dr. Page found patients with different ethnic backgrounds all benefited from this combination of foods.[3]

Another dentist, Dr. William Donald Kelley also balanced the autonomic nervous system with food. Dr. Kelley developed pancreatic cancer in 1962 and was given weeks to live; however, by applying his research in nutrition, he extended his own life until 2003. Dr. Kelley's program had 10 diets with different combinations of plant and animal-based foods as well as raw and cooked foods to balance an individual's autonomic nervous system. The right diet for each person is the one that balances his or her autonomic nervous system.[4] This is why some people feel better on a plant-based diet while others need animal protein to feel their best. The bottom line is that no person can be healthy eating a diet consisting predominantly of processed food.

Today's researchers continue to unlock the mysteries of the autonomic nervous system. Imbalances in the autonomic nervous system can be identified in a noninvasive way by looking at heart rate variability (known as HRV) which is a measure of the variation in time between each heartbeat. Low HRV suggests one is in fight or flight mode whereas high HRV suggests a rest and digest state. Research shows low HRV is associated with chronic disease such as cardiovascular disease and depression. HRV can be measured and analyzed with a chest strap monitor and smartphone app.

Osteopathic physician, Dr. Patrick Nemechek has dedicated his career to studying autonomic dysfunction and its role in chronic disease, especially neurological diseases such as autism and developmental disorders. Dr. Nemechek has developed The Nemechek Protocol to restore neurological function. He believes childhood developmental disorders arise from brain inflammation from overgrowth of intestinal bacteria (the kind of bacteria that thrive on simple carbohydrates found in processed food). Dr. Nemechek's protocol balances intestinal bacteria decreasing inflammation both in the brain and body, and also restores the balance of omega-6 and omega-3 fatty acids in the body.[5]

Sources of omega-3 fatty acids include fatty fish such as salmon as well as plant sources such as chia and flax seed. These fatty acids are essential because they cannot be made by our bodies. We must consume them in our diets. They are also essential because they are a vital part of many structures of our body such as the cell membrane. Omega-3 fatty acids are anti-inflammatory. Omega-6 fatty acids are found in vegetable oils such as corn oil and soybean oil, common ingredients in many processed foods. Sadly, many people consume no anti-inflammatory omega-3 fatty acids in their diets and instead consume large quantities of pro-inflammatory omega-6 fatty acids leading to the myriad of degenerative diseases common today.

Would you like to see for yourself how changing your diet improves your health? Follow these steps:

1. Drink water (not soda, fruit juice, or any other drinks sweetened with sugar or artificial sweeteners).

2. Eliminate highly processed foods containing flour and sugar.

3. Eat a variety of fresh, whole, nutrient dense foods that meet nutritional requirements for human beings. One easy way to do this is to add vegetables in all colors of the rainbow into your diet.

4. Think about where your ancestors came from and what foods they would have eaten generations ago before processed food was available. These foods will likely be good for you too.

5. Choose foods that must be thoroughly chewed and chew them thoroughly. If you feel like you need to drink a lot of water while you are eating, it is likely that you are not chewing your food thoroughly enough.

6. Recognize the need for special nutrition throughout various stages of life, preconception through advanced years.

Good facial structure will develop when human beings thoroughly chew a variety of nutrient-dense whole foods containing all nutrients essential for bone growth and development. Good facial structure means that there is room for all teeth including the wisdom teeth. The nasal passages are large enough for optimal flow of air into the nose and sinuses. The tongue rests in the roof of the mouth ensuring nasal breathing and a functional swallow. The autonomic nervous system is perfectly balanced bringing excellent health to the entire body. This was the normal structure and function for all human beings before processed food and is illustrated in the case of these two Australian Aborigines photographed by Dr. Price. These boys are brothers, the first conceived when the parents were living in their native environment eating native foods, and the second after they moved to a reservation and were eating processed foods provided by the government. By now, I'm sure you will immediately notice the difference in the shape of the dental arches.

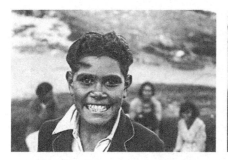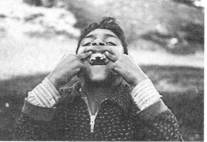

These same principles of nature hold true today. The two girls in the following photographs are sisters when each was about 4-1/2 years of age. They are my daughters. I was not healthy during my pregnancy with Alyssa, on the left, due to yet-to-be diagnosed digestive problems and I ate mostly processed food because it was all I could tolerate. Thanks to fresh, whole food, I underwent tremendous healing between pregnancies and continued to eat highly nutritious food throughout my pregnancy with Veronica, on the right. We can see the difference in their teeth. There are no spaces between Alyssa's teeth. At the time, I thought "what beautiful straight teeth she has." Little did I know this would not last as she grew.

As of this writing, Alyssa is now 3-½ years into the ALF treatment process and has space for all of her permanent teeth. She completed nine months of myofunctional therapy. Veronica is opening up to the idea of myofunctional therapy. Both girls eat plenty of fresh, whole food and receive regular osteopathic treatments. Here are their pictures today:

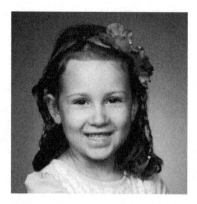 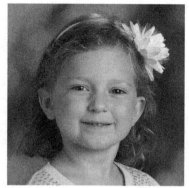

This experience is not unique to my family. Parents in my practice have also noticed that as their own health improves, their children's facial structure and overall health improves as well. Some have observed the reverse. As they work through the ALF treatment process with their children, their own health problems diminish and they are better able to achieve their own health goals.

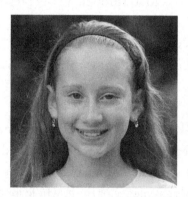 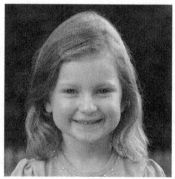

Processed food negatively impacts facial structure. As you have learned in the discussion of osteopathic principles, structure and function are reciprocally interrelated. With the change in facial structure comes change in function, namely mouth breathing and dysfunctional swallow. Then we have an unbalanced autonomic nervous system leading to poor overall health. This is the state of the human being today and the reason why failure to thrive, ADHD, bed-wetting, anxiety, sleep apnea, digestive problems, high blood pressure and so many other conditions are prevalent today.

Fortunately, it doesn't have to be this way. Instead, with osteopathy, the ALF appliance, myofunctional therapy, and a nutrient dense whole food diet, we can guide the structure of the mouth and rehabilitate function to return to the way it was created to be. Through epigenetics, there is hope future generations can once again experience the joy of excellent health. Along with this level of health comes the physical, emotional and spiritual resilience necessary to thrive in today's world. I am blessed to offer my own children, and my patients, this opportunity.

CHAPTER 8

Conclusion

This book was written with the intent of creating a paradigm shift within the perspective of traditional orthodontics from a "teeth focus" to a "whole body health focus." I hope the information presented creates openness to opportunities to dive deeper with wonder, curiosity, and collaboration as we progress into "forward-focused orthodontics." This transformation starts with the question of what creates crooked teeth. What is the etiology of malocclusions? The answer of the past has been "your mouth is too small for your teeth. You must have received the genes of your mouth from your mother and your teeth genes from your father." This situation creates a small mouth with large teeth. The solution of the past has been to remove the teeth to create more space for the teeth at the expense of the volume of space within the mouth, thus limiting our airway and creating a head forward posture.

We now know that the answer of the "mismatch" between size of palate and teeth is explained by the concept of epigenetics, which explains how genes are activated by the environment (i.e. function). As humans we share 96% of the same genes. Which genes are activated to create a physiological change depends on the environment we are exposed to. Our environment creates our functions and thus determines our structure. It is the intra and extra oral functions of nasal breathing, a functional swallow, and chewing pattern that create the structure of the face. Our genetics provide the substance available to use to manifest our structures. When these underlying dysfunctions are treated at the same time teeth are moved, a whole body integration is created with no need of a lifetime oral retainer to "hold" the treatment. The underlying dysfunctions have been addressed and the teeth position will express the integrated functions, thus maintaining the space needed for optimal function and health. Simply put, malocclusions are the symptoms of an imbalance in the body function and structure.

The concept of biotensegrity may also lay a foundation in understanding the integration of the body as one functioning unit. The biotensegrity model explains the body as a complex system moving in compensatory balancing motion with constant tensile forces of compression/decompression to create a stable functioning unit of biology. Any change in one area of the body will create compensations in another in order to maintain the overall homeostasis and balance. As the dental occlusion changes, the compensatory effects are distributed through the entire body. With a "forward health focused" approach to changes in the dental occlusion, there is a potential for healing pathologies previously considered to be non-dental in origin.

Thixotropy, perhaps another new concept, is a property of colloidal tissue, a basic substrate of the human body. Thixotropy explains that a substance can react as a liquid or solid depending on the level of force the substance comes into contact with. Rapid, forceful changes create restrictions in motion in the human body and potential disintegration of the parts of the body. For example, a rapid forceful change in the position of the teeth can have an effect on the position of the mandible, affecting the temporal bone motion. As discussed in Chapter 6, this potential limitation of motion within the craniofacial cervical complex could have an effect on the lymphatic and venous drainage of the brain, leading to suboptimal functioning. A softer slower process (the ALF Approach) allows the body to compensate and integrate the changes without creating tissue compression and restrictions to motion. When the dental occlusion is altered with the limited perspective of a "teeth focused" approach, the strain patterns of the craniofacial cervical complex (which are part of the etiology of the malocclusion) can be "locked" into a dysfunction. This dysfunction of the structure and function is reactivated every time the teeth contact, creating a lifetime dysfunction that can become challenging and sometimes impossible to transform without changing the position of the teeth. As enamel is the hardest substance in the body and the dental occlusion is the largest "joint" in the body, this dictates the position and function of the craniofacial cervical complex as well as potentially the entire structure of the body. With an osteopathic and myofunctional collaborative approach, the underlying etiologies of the malocclusion can be integrated to allow the body to function as an optimally functional unit of health. The osteopathic treatments can engage the restricted compressed areas in order to integrate them back into the body as a whole, thus the body can function properly together as a functional unit of motion. Motion is the key element in biotensegrity, thixotropy, osteopathy, and the ALF Approach.

The ALF Approach is a team approach to treating malocclusions as a symptom of craniofacial cervical dysfunctions. The team includes the ALF-trained orthodontist/dentist, ALF-trained cranial osteopathic physician, and ALF-trained myofunctional therapist. Each one of these professions provides an essential component of the treatment. The ALF appliances were created within the "womb of osteopathy" and adhere to the principles of osteopathy. The team members in the ALF Approach need to become educated to follow these principles throughout the course of treatment. The ALF appliances are "health appliances" and are not simply an orthodontics appliance. They act as a biometric tongue to the base of the cranium. In this way the cranial rhythmic impulse is augmented, the cranial base is stimulated to elongate, the lip seal nasal breathing reflex is activated, and thus the head begins to move backwards, re-aligning itself over the cervical vertebrae. This changes the position of the body and restores physiological motion and health.

Key points to take away from this book

1. Form follows Function.

2. Function is motion and motion is Health.

3. The major functions that grow a face are nasal breathing, functional swallow, and functional chewing.

4. Birth trauma that compresses the occiput (which is in four pieces at birth) and potentially the cranial nerves 9-12 affect facial growth and development as well as digestion.

5. The human body grows into a form to maximize survival, which is our "airway."

6. Teeth placement are a result of the position of the upper and lower jaw within the craniofacial complex and the pattern of contraction of the intra and extra orofacial muscles.

7. The cranial bones have a subtle motion allowing for optimal central nervous system venous and lymphatic drainage.

8. The resting position of the tongue in the upper palate is the major influence that creates the shape and size of the upper palate and midface growth.

9. Facial growth and development is driven by epigenetics.

10. We are losing our forward facial growth secondary to our lack of mandibular stimulation to chewing hard food. If you don't use it, you lose it!

11. Our bodies are one integrating, unifying, complex system held together by biotensegrity.

12. Our tissues respond to a hard fast compression with a hardening, and a soft slow engagement with a softening. Our tissues follow the principle of thixotropy.

13. Trauma and injuries can create soft tissue compressive forces that affect long term compressibility of tissue and thus function.

14. Lymphatic and venous drainage are motion-dependent systems.

15. The brain drains toxins out at night while we are sleeping.

16. The brain toxins drain out through a space between the temporal and occipital bones into the deep cervical lymph nodes that lie behind the front neck muscles.

17. Compromise to the motion of the temporal and/or occipital bone can create a less than optimal brain drain.

18. An anterior tongue thrust swallowing pattern (immature swallow) does not stimulate pressure to the base of the cranium to stimulate growth of the basicranium, augment the cranial motion, drain the sinuses and middle ear, and develop the mid-face.

19. Head forward posture can be a result of a deficient "airway," increased technology time, and an inhibition of core muscle development in our infants with the overuse of infant seats and other devices.

20. Head posture affects the position of the upper and lower jaw, and vice versa.

21. The mandible is a super-cool bone. We need it for survival so it has to have many adaptable capacities to grow with epigenetic influences.

22. The position and motion of the temporal bone is missed by most dentists treating temporomandibular disorder (TMD).

23. Most cranial osteopaths do not know how to assess intra-oral function to assess the dental occlusion's effect on cranial motion.

24. The ALF is a super-cool dental appliance. It is an osteopathic, myofunctional, orthopedic, and orthodontic appliance.

25. All dentists using the ALF need to take courses in how to treat with the ALF, and all osteopaths treating with the ALF need to take courses in how to treat with the appliance and communicate with the dentist.

26. Myofunctional therapy is essential therapy in the ALF Approach.

27. The goal of the ALF Approach is to restore and rehabilitate the physiological function of the craniofacial cervical complex (head, face, neck).

28. The body is a functioning unit.

29. Structure and function are reciprocally interrelated.

30. The vagus is an important nerve for health. It can be impinged in many places, which can affect optimal functioning of the nerve, as it is the longest nerve in the body.

31. The functioning of the vagus can affect emotional fight/flight trauma responses.

32. Osteopathic treatments can help treat vagal nerve dysfunctions.

Resources

Where to find ALF team members

ALF-trained dentists

AEI (ALF Educational Institute) lists ALF-certified dentists who have completed the collaborative and integrative ALF training through AEI, which includes a practical and written exam. Tasha Turzo, DO, James Bronson, DDS, and Kathy Winslow, RDH, are the faculty for this extensive and highly educational program. https://alfeducationalinstitute.com/alf-certified-dentists/

Ljuba Lemke, DMD, lists ALF-trained dentists who have completed her online courses: www.alternativeorthodontics.com

InterFace by Dr. Darick Nordstrom (creator of the ALF) lists ALF-trained dentists and osteopaths who have a membership to his online webinar: https://alfinterface.academy/

Dr. Tasha Turzo's website lists ALF-trained dentists who have completed the collaborative and integrative ALF training through AEI (ALF Educational Institute): www.drtashaturzo.com

ALF-trained cranial osteopathic physicians

Dr. Tasha Turzo's website lists cranial osteopathic physicians who have completed the AEI (ALF Educational Institute) residency program: www.drtashaturzo.com

InterFace by Dr. Darick Nordstrom (creator of the ALF) lists ALF-trained osteopaths who have a membership to his online webinar: https://alfinterface.academy/

Osteopathic physicians in the US

This website lists osteopaths who have specialized in cranial osteopathy. When looking for a physician, make sure that they have a ranking of at least 90% next to their name, as this indicates the amount of cranial osteopathy they practice in their clinics. A star by their name indicates that they have passed the proficiency exam in cranial osteopathy. https://cranialacademy.org/find-a-physician/

This website lists osteopaths specializing in neuromuscular medicine and osteopathy. Some will be proficient in cranial osteopathy and some will not. https://www.academyofosteopathy.org/find-an-osteopathic-physician

International biodynamic-trained DOs

This website lists international practitioners who have studied with Dr. James Jealous and/or his faculty in the field of biodynamic osteopathy, which is the study of Dr. Sutherland's work in his later years of practicing osteopathy. Biodynamics offers insight and skills to treat the patient from a fluid perspective. https://www.jamesjealous.com/additional-resources/physician-directory/

Orofacial myofunctional therapists

The best-known associations for training in orofacial myofunctional therapy are:

IAOM (International Association of Orofacial Myology) – member directory: http://orofacialmyologist.org/

AAMS (Academy of Applied Myofunctional Sciences) – member directory: https://www.myofunctionaltherapists.com/

Dr. Tasha Turzo's website lists OMFTs who have completed the AEI (ALF Educational Institute) residency program: www.drtashaturzo.com

References

Introduction

[1] http://portlandtmjclinic.com/etiology/chapter-4

Chapter 1

[1] Miyawaki, S., Tanimoto, Y., Araki, Y., Katayama, A., Fujii, A., & Takano-Yamamoto, T. (2003). Association Between Nocturnal Bruxism and Gastroesophageal Reflux. *Sleep, 26*(7), 939-940.

[2] Mokhlesi, B. (2003). Clinical Implications of Gastroesophageal Reflux Disease and Swallowing Dysfunction in COPD. *American Journal of Respiratory Medicine, 2*(2), 117–121.

[3] Close L. G. (2002). Laryngopharyngeal manifestations of reflux: diagnosis and therapy. *European Journal of Gastroenterology & Hepatology,* 14 Suppl 1, S23–S27.

[4] Teramoto, S., Kume, H., & Ouchi, Y. (2002). Nocturnal Gastroesophageal Reflux. *Chest, 122*(6), 2266-2267.

[5] Orr, W. C. (2002). Sleep-Related Breathing Disorders. *Chest, 121*(1), 8–11.

[6] Calhoun, W. J. (2003). Nocturnal Asthma. *Chest, 123*(3), 399S-405S.

[7] Issing, W. J. (2003). Gastroesophageal Reflux – a common illness? *Laryngo-Rhino-Otologie, 82*(2), 118–122.

[8] McBratney-Owen, B., Iseki, S., Bamforth, S. D., Olsen, B. R., & Morriss-Kay, G. M. (2008). Development and tissue origins of the mammalian cranial base. *Developmental Biology, 322*(1), 121–132.

[9] Blechschmidt, E. (Author), Freeman, B. (Editor) (2004). *The Ontogenetic Basis of Human Anatomy: A Biodynamic Approach to Development from Conception to Birth* (1st ed.). North Atlantic Books. p.142.

[10] Perronneaud-Ferré R. (1989). Ostéopathie cranio-pelvienne. La technique des blocs. Aix en Provence: Editions de Verlaque.[French]– Lignon A. 1989. Le puzzle cranien. Aix en Provence: Editions de Verlaque. [French] – Upledger JE, Vredevoogd JD. 1996.Terapia craniosacrale. Teoria e metodo. Como: Red Edizioni. [Italian] – Sutherland WG. 2002. Enseignements

dans la science de l'ostéopathie. Fort Worth, Texas: Sutherland Cranial Teaching Foundation. Inc. [French]

[11] Da Silva, J.T.; Farbiarz, J.L. (2016). O pensamento de Buckminster Fuller e o LILD, PUC-Rio. 2016 (2007-2008). http://pdf.blucher.com.br.s3-sa-east-1.amazonaws.com/designproceedings/ped2016/0170.pdf

[12] https://thehealinglotus.ca/lotus-notes/what-you-need-to-know-about-tensegrity-and-the-human-structure

[13] https://www.innerbody.com/image/musc06.html

[14] https://en.wikipedia.org/wiki/Time-dependent_viscosity

[15] https://en.wikipedia.org/wiki/Time-dependent_viscosity#cite_note-1

Chapter 2

[1] Crow, W. T., King, H. H., Patterson, R. M., & Giuliano, V. (2009). Assessment of calvarial structure motion by MRI. *Osteopathic Medicine and Primary Care*, 3(1), 8.

[2] Ueno, Toshiaki, et al. (1998) Noninvasive measurement of pulsatile intracranial pressure using ultrasound. *Intracranial Pressure and Neuromonitoring in Brain Injury*. Springer, Vienna. 66-69.

[3] Moskalenko, Y. E., Kravchenko, T. I., Gaidar, B. V., Vainshtein, G. B., Semernya, V. N., Maiorova, N. F., & Mitrofanov, V. F. (1999). Periodic mobility of cranial bones in humans. *Human Physiology*, 25(1), 51-58

[4] Heifetz, M. D., & Weiss, M. (1981). Detection of skull expansion with increased intracranial pressure. *Journal of Neurosurgery*, 55(5), 811–812.

[5] Gard, G. (2009). An investigation into the regulation of intra-cranial pressure and its influence upon the surrounding cranial bones. *Journal of Bodywork and Movement Therapies*, 13(3), 246–254.

[6] Heisey, S. R., & Adams, T. (1993). Role of Cranial Bone Mobility in Cranial Compliance. *Neurosurgery*, 33(5), 869–877.

[7] Heisey, S.R., &, Adams, T. (1995). A two compartment model for cranial compliance. *Journal of the American Osteopathic Association*, (95)547. https://www.iahe.com/docs/articles/Cranial-Sutures-and-Sutural-Movement-Resources.pdf

[8] Adams, T., Heisey, R.S., Smith, M.C., Briner, B.J. (1992). Parietal bone mobility in the anesthetized cat. *Journal of the American Osteopathic Association*, 92(5):599-622

[9] Ballard, R.E., Wilson, M., Hargens, A.R., et al. (1996) Noninvasive measurement of intracranial volume and pressure using ultrasound. *American Institute of Aeronautics and Astronautics Life Sciences and Space Medicine Conference. Book of Abstracts*, pp. 76-77, Houston, TX.

[10] Ueno, T., Ballard, R.E., Cantrell, J.H., Yost, W.T., Hargens, A.R. (1996) Noninvasive estimation of pulsatile intracranial pressure using ultrasound. *Research & Technology: Human Exploration and Development of Space Enterprise: Technology Applications to Human Health*. NASA Ames Research Center.

[11] Ueno, T., Ballard, R.E., Shuer, L.M., Yost, W.T., Cantrell, J.H., Hargens, A.R. (1997) Ultrasonic measurement of intracranial pressure waveforms. *Aeronautics & Space Transportation Technology Enterprise*. NASA Ames

[12] Ueno, T., Ballard, R. E., Shuer, L. M., Cantrell, J. H., Yost, W. T., & Hargens, A. R. (1998). Noninvasive Measurement of Pulsatile Intracranial Pressure Using Ultrasound. *Intracranial Pressure and Neuromonitoring in Brain Injury*, 95, 66–69.

[13] Hargens, A.R.(1999) Noninvasive intracranial pressure (ICP) measurement. *Space Physiology Laboratory*. http://spacephysiology.arc.nasa.gov/projects/icp.html

[14] Crow, W. T., King, H. H., Patterson, R. M., & Giuliano, V. (2009). Assessment of calvarial structure motion by MRI. *Osteopathic Medicine and Primary Care*, 3(1), 8.

[15] Oleski, S. L., Smith, G. H., & Crow, W. T. (2002). Radiographic Evidence of Cranial Bone Mobility. *CRANIO®*, 20(1), 34–38.

[16] Michael, D.K., Retzlaff, E.W. (1975) A preliminary study of cranial bone movement in the squirrel monkey. *Journal of the American Osteopathic Association*, 74, 866-869

[17] Adams, T., Heisey, R.S., Smith, M.C., Briner, B.J. (1992) Parietal bone mobility in the anesthetized cat. *Journal of the American Osteopathic Association*, 92(5): 599-622.

[18] Moskalenko, Y.E., Frymann, V.M., Weinstein, G.B., Semernya, V.N., Kravchenko, T.I., Markovets, S.P., … Maiorova, N.S. (2001) Slow rhythmic oscillations within the human cranium phenomenology, origin, and informational significance. *Human Physiology*, 27(2): 171-178.

Chapter 3

[1] Frymann, V., DO, FAAO (1997). The Expanding Osteopathic Concept,

Development of Cranial Bones, p. 54

[2] https://cranialacademy.org/

[3] https://en.wikipedia.org/wiki/Jugular_foramen_syndrome

[4] Erol, F. S., Kaplan, M., Kavakli, A., & Ozveren, M. F. (2005). Jugular foramen syndrome caused by choleastatoma. *Clinical Neurology and Neurosurgery*, 107(4), 342–346.

[5] Quinones-Hinojosa, Alfredo, ed. (2012). *Schmidek and Sweet Indications, Methods and Results (Expert Consult – Online and Print)* (6th ed.). London: Elsevier Health Sciences. p. 2337. ISBN 9781455723287.

Chapter 4

[1] Wadsworth et al, 1998

[2] Stahl, F., Grabowski, R., Gaebel, M., & Kundt, G. (2007). Relationship between Occlusal Findings and Orofacial Myofunctional Status in Primary and Mixed Dentition. *Journal of Orofacial Orthopedics / Fortschritte Der Kieferorthopädie*, 68(2), 74–90.

[3] Domínguez-Ortega, L., & de Vicente-Colomina, A. (2006). Trastorno por déficit de atención con hiperactividad y alteraciones del sueño. *Medicina Clínica*, 126(13), 500–506.

[4] Gozal, D. (1998). Sleep-Disordered Breathing and School Performance in Children. *Pediatrics*, 102(3), 616–620.

[5] Weissbluth, M., Davis, A.T., Poncher, J., & Reiff, J. (1983). Signs of Airway Obstruction During Sleep and Behavioral, Developmental, and Academic Problems. *Journal of Developmental & Behavioral Pediatrics*, 4(2), 119–121.

[6] Leng, Y., McEvoy, C. T., Allen, I. E., & Yaffe, K. (2017). Association of Sleep-Disordered Breathing With Cognitive Function and Risk of Cognitive Impairment. *JAMA Neurology*, 74(10), 1237.

[7] da Silva-Júnior, F. P., do Prado, G. F., Barbosa, E. R., Tufik, S., & Togeiro, S. M. (2014). Sleep Disordered Breathing in Parkinson's Disease: A Critical Appraisal. *Sleep Medicine Reviews*, 18(2), 173–178.

[8] Huang, Y.-S., Hsu, S.-C., Guilleminault, C., & Chuang, L.-C. (2019). Myofunctional Therapy. *Sleep Medicine Clinics*, 14(1), 135–142.

[9] Guilleminault, C., Huang, Y. S., Monteyrol, P. J., Sato, R., Quo, S., & Lin, C. H. (2013). Critical role of myofascial reeducation in pediatric sleep-disordered breathing. *Sleep Medicine*, 14(6), 518–525.

[10] Moeller, J. L., Paskay, L. C., & Gelb, M. L. (2014b). Myofunctional Therapy. *Sleep Medicine Clinics*, 9(2), 235–243.

[11] Villa, M. P., Evangelisti, M., Martella, S., Barreto, M., & Del Pozzo, M. (2017). Can myofunctional therapy increase tongue tone and reduce symptoms in children with sleep-disordered breathing? *Sleep and Breathing*, 21(4), 1025–1032.

[12] Cooper, A. (2010). Orofacial Myology and Myofunctional Therapy for Sleep Related Breathing Disorders. *Sleep Medicine Clinics*, 5(1), 109–113.

[13] Camacho, M., Certal, V., Abdullatif, J., Zaghi, S., Ruoff, C. M., Capasso, R., & Kushida, C. A. (2015). Myofunctional Therapy to Treat Obstructive Sleep Apnea: A Systematic Review and Meta-analysis. *Sleep*, 38(5), 669–675.

[14] Frey, L., Green, S., Fabbie, P., Hockenbury, D., Foran, M., & Elder, K. (2014). The Essential Role of the COM in the Management of Sleep-Disordered Breathing: A Literature Review and Discussion. *The International Journal of Orofacial Myology*, 40, 42–55.

[15] Lieberman, D. E. (2011). *The Evolution of the Human Head*, Harvard University Press.

[16] Enlow, D.H., Hans, M.G. (1996). *Essentials of Facial Growth*, Needham Press, p.2

[17] Van Der Klaauw, C. J. (1952). Size and Position of the Functional Components of the Skull. a Contribution To the Knowledge of the Architecture of the Skull, Based On Data in the Literature. *Archives Néerlandaises de Zoologie*, 9(1), 1–556.

[18] Moss, M. L. (1964). Vertical growth of the human face. *American Journal of Orthodontics*, 50(5), 359–376.

[19] Moss-Salentijn, L. (1997). Melvin L. Moss and the Functional Matrix. *Journal of Dental Research*, 76(12), 1814–1817.

[20] Gozala, D. & Kheirandish-Gozal, L. (2007) *Current Opinion in Pulmonary Medicine* 13:505-509

[21] Bonuck, Karen, Freeman, K., Chervin, R. D., & Xu, L. (2012). Sleep-Disordered Breathing in a Population-Based Cohort: Behavioral Outcomes at 4 and 7 Years. *Pediatrics*, 129(4), e857–e865.

[22] Defabians (2000) Ankyloglossia and its influence on maxillary and mandibular development (A seven year follow-up case report) *Functional Orthodontics*, 17(4): 25-33

[23] Winslow, K.L. (Interview), Lee, C. (2015). Improving Overall Health Through Orofacial Myofunctional Therapy, *CDHA Journal*, 32(1), 23.

[24] Guimarães, K. C., Drager, L. F., Genta, P. R., Marcondes, B. F., & Lorenzi-Filho, G. (2009). Effects of Oropharyngeal Exercises on Patients with Moderate Obstructive Sleep Apnea Syndrome. *American Journal of Respiratory and Critical Care Medicine*, 179(10), 962–966.

[25] Simon, P.M., Landry, S.H., Leiter, J.C.. (20020. Respiratory control during sleep. in: Lee-Chiong TL, Sateia MJ, Carskadon MA, editors. *Sleep Medicine*. Philadelphia: Hanley & Beifus; p. 41-51

[26] Lee, S.-Y., Guilleminault, C., Chiu, H.-Y., & Sullivan, S. S. (2015). Mouth breathing, "nasal disuse," and pediatric sleep-disordered breathing. *Sleep and Breathing*, 19(4), 1257–1264.

[27] Guimarães, K. C., Drager, L. F., Genta, P. R., Marcondes, B. F., & Lorenzi-Filho, G. (2009b). Effects of Oropharyngeal Exercises on Patients with Moderate Obstructive Sleep Apnea Syndrome. *American Journal of Respiratory and Critical Care Medicine*, 179(10), 962–966.

[28] Angle, E. H. (1907). *Treatment of Malocclusion of the Teeth: Angle's System* (7th ed.). Philadelphia, Pennsylvania: White Dental Manufacturing Co.

[29] Suzuki, H., Watanabe, A., Akihiro, Y., Takao, M., Ikematsu, T., Kimoto, S., … Kawara, M. (2013). Pilot study to assess the potential of oral myofunctional therapy for improving respiration during sleep. *Journal of Prosthodontic Research*, 57(3), 195–199.

[30] Guilleminault, C., Huang, Y. S., Monteyrol, P. J., Sato, R., Quo, S., & Lin, C. H. (2013). Critical role of myofascial reeducation in pediatric sleep-disordered breathing. *Sleep Medicine*, 14(6), 518–525.

[31] Camacho, M., Certal, V., Abdullatif, J., Zaghi, S., Ruoff, C. M., Capasso, R., & Kushida, C. A. (2015). Myofunctional Therapy to Treat Obstructive Sleep Apnea: A Systematic Review and Meta-analysis. *Sleep*, 38(5), 669–675.

[32] Vandenplas, Y., Denayer, E., Vandenbossche, T., Vermet, L., Hauser, B., DeSchepper, J., & Engelen, A. (2008). Osteopathy may decrease obstructive apnea in infants: a pilot study. *Osteopathic Medicine and Primary Care*, 2(1), 8.

[33] Mao, J. J., Wang, X., & Kopher, R. A. (2003). Biomechanics of craniofacial sutures: Orthopedic implications. *Angle Orthodontics*, 73(2), 128–135.

[34] Price, W. A. (2009). *Nutrition and Physical Degeneration* (8th ed.). Lemon Grove, CA: Price-Pottenger Nutrition Foundation.

[35] Kahn, S., & Ehrlich, P. R. (2018). *Jaws: The Story of a Hidden Epidemic* (1st ed.). Stanford University Press.

[36] Price, Westin A. (2006). *Nutrition and Physical Degeneration* (7th ed.). Price-Pottenger Nutrition Foundation. pp. 256-281.

[37] Rappaport, K. (2015). The Developmental Progression of Eating Skills Identification of Early Feeding Issues. *CDHA Journal*, 32(1), 6-11.

[38] Ung, N., Koenig, J., Shapiro, P. A., Shapiro, G., & Trask, G. (1990). A quantitative assessment of respiratory patterns and their effects on dentofacial development. *American Journal of Orthodontics and Dentofacial Orthopedics*, 98(6), 523–532.

[39] Al Ali, A., Richmond, S., Popat, H., Playle, R., Pickles, T., Zhurov, A. I., … Bonuck, K. (2015). The influence of snoring, mouth breathing and apnoea on facial morphology in late childhood: a three-dimensional study. *BMJ Open*, 5(9), e009027.

[40] Guilleminault, C., & S Sullivan, S. (2014). Towards Restoration of Continuous Nasal Breathing as the Ultimate Treatment Goal in Pediatric Obstructive Sleep Apnea. *Enliven: Pediatrics and Neonatal Biology*, 01(01).

[41] Imbard, A., Benoist, J.-F., & Blom, H. (2013). Neural Tube Defects, Folic Acid and Methylation. *International Journal of Environmental Research and Public Health*, 10(9), 4352–4389.

[42] Huang, Y., Quo, S., Berkowski, J. A., & Guilleminault, C. (2015). Short Lingual Frenulum and Obstructive Sleep Apnea in Children. *Int J Pediatr Res*, 1:003

[43] Baxter DMD MS, R. (2018). *Tongue-Tied: How a Tiny String Under the Tongue Impacts Nursing, Speech, Feeding, and More.* Alabama Tongue-Tie Center. p.201-202

[44] Castelo, P. M., Gaviao, M. B. D., Pereira, L. J., & Bonjardim, L. R. (2005). Relationship between oral parafunctional/nutritive sucking habits and temporomandibular joint dysfunction in primary dentition. *International Journal of Paediatric Dentistry*, 15(1), 29–36.

[45] Ferreira, C. L. P., Machado, B. C. Z., Borges, C. G. P., Rodrigues Da Silva, M. A. M., Sforza, C., & De Felício, C. M. (2014). Impaired orofacial motor functions on chronic temporomandibular disorders. *Journal of Electromyography and Kinesiology*, 24(4), 565–571.

[46] Hruska Jr., R.J. (1997). Influences of dysfunctional respiratory mechanics on orofacial pain. *Dental Clinics of North America* 41, 211-227

[47] Huang, Y.-S., & Guilleminault, C. (2013). Pediatric Obstructive Sleep Apnea and the Critical Role of Oral-Facial Growth: Evidence. *Frontiers in Neurology*, 3.

[48] Galland, B., Spruyt, K., Dawes, P., McDowall, P. S., Elder, D., & Schaughency, E. (2015). Sleep Disordered Breathing and Academic Performance: A Meta-analysis. *Pediatrics*, 136(4), e934–e946.

[49] Gozal, D., & Kheirandish-Gozal, L. (2007). Neurocognitive and behavioral morbidity in children with sleep disorders. *Current Opinion in Pulmonary Medicine*, 13(6), 505–509.

[50] Bonuck, K., Rao, T., & Xu, L. (2012). Pediatric Sleep Disorders and Special Educational Need at 8 Years: A Population-Based Cohort Study. *Pediatrics*, 130(4), 634–642.

[51] Winslow, K.L. (Interview), Lee, C. (2015). Improving Overall Health Through Orofacial Myofunctional Therapy, *CDHA Journal*, 32(1), 23

[52] Winslow, K.L. (Interview), Lee, C. (2015). Improving Overall Health Through Orofacial Myofunctional Therapy, *CDHA Journal*, 32(1), 23.

[53] Proffit, W. R., Fields, Jr., H. W., & Sarver, D. M. (2006). *Contemporary Orthodontics* (4th ed.). St. Louis, Missouri: Mosby.

Chapter 5

[1] Scoppa, F., & Pirino, A. (2019). Is there a relationship between body posture and tongue posture? Glosso-Postural syndrome between myth and Reality. *Acta Medica Mediterranea*, 35, 1903.

[2] Zafar H. (2000). Integrated jaw and neck function in man: studies of mandibular and head-neck movements during jaw opening-closing tasks. Swedish Dental Journal Suppl, 143:1-41.

[3] Eriksson PO, Haggman-Henrikson B, Nordh E, Zafar H. (2000). Coordinated mandibular and head-neck movements during rhythmic jaw activities in man. Journal of Dental Research, 79:1378-1384.

[4] Varrela J. (1990). Occurrence of malocclusion in attritive environment: a study of a skull sample from southwest Finland. *European Journal of Oral Science*, 98:242-247.

[5] Sakaguchi, K., Mehta, N. R., Abdallah, E. F., Forgione, A. G., Hirayama, H., Kawasaki, T., & Yokoyama, A. (2007). Examination of the

Relationship Between Mandibular Position and Body Posture. CRANIO®, 25(4), 237–249.

[6] Beyron H. (1964). Occlusal relations and mastication in Australian Aborigines. *Acta Odontologica Scandinavica*, 22:597-678.

[7] Angel JL. (1948). Factors in temporomandibular joint form. *American Journal of Anatomy*, 83:223-246.

[8] Moffett BC, Johnson LC, McCabe JB, Askew HC. (1964). Articular remodelling in the adult temporomandibular joint. *American Journal of Anatomy*, 115:119-142.

[9] Woda A, Pionchon P, Palla S. (2001). Regulation of mandibular postures: mechanisms and clinical implications. *Critical Reviews in Oral Biology and Medicine*; 12(2):166-78.

[10] Solow B, Sandham A. (2002). Craniocervical posture: a factor in the development and function of the dentofacial structures. *European Journal of Orthodontics*, 24:447-456.

[11] Springate SD. (2012). A re-investigation of the relationship between head posture and craniofacial growth. *European Journal of Orthodontics*, 34(4):397-409.

[12] Choi J-K. (1992). A study of the effects of maximal voluntary clenching on the tooth contact points and masticatory muscle activities in patients with temporomandibular disorders. *Journal of Craniomandibular Disorder Facial Oral Pain* 6:41-46.

[13] Zafar H. (2002). Integrated jaw and neck function in man: studies of mandibular and head-neck movements during jaw opening-closing tasks. *Swedish Dental Journal Suppl.* 143:1-41.

[14] Tecco S, Tete S, Festa F. (2010). Electromyographic evaluation of masticatory, neck, and trunk muscle activity in patients with posterior crossbites. *European Journal of Orthodontics*, 32(6):747-752.

[15] Darling DW, Kraus S, Glasheen-Wray MB. (1984). Relationship of head posture and the rest position of the mandible. *Journal of Prosthetic Dentistry*, 52:111-115.

[16] Elgoyhen JC, Moyers RE, McNamara JA, Riolo MI. (1972). Craniofacial adaptation to protrusive function in young rhesus monkeys. *American Journal of Orthodontics*, 62(5):469-480.

[17] Goldstein DF, Kraus SL, Williams WB, Glasheen-Wray M. (1984).

Influence of cervical posture on mandibular movement. *Journal of Prosthetic Dentistry*, 52:421-426.

[18] Harvold EP, Tomer BS, Vargervik K, Chierici G. (1981). Primate experiments on oral respiration. *American Journal of Orthodontics*, 79(4):359-372.

[19] Helm S, Prydso U. (1979). Prevalence of malocclusion in medieval and modern Danes contrasted. *European Journal of Oral Sciences*, 87(2):91-97.

[20] Koidis P. (1986). Influence of postural position on occlusal contact strain patterns. *Journal of Dental Research*, 65 (special issue abstr 178):189.

[21] Maeda N, Sakaguchi K, Mehta NR, et al. (2011). Effects of experimental leg length discrepancies on body posture and dental occlusion. *Journal of Craniomandibular Practice*, 29(3):194-203.

[22] Marsan G, Oztas E, Cura N, Kuvat SV, et al. (2010). Changes in head posture and hyoid bone position in Turkish class 3 patients after mandibular setback surgery. *Journal of Craniomaxillofacial Surgery*, 38(2):113-121.

[23] McClean LF, Brenman HS, Friedman MG. (1973). Effects of changing body position on dental occlusion. *Journal of Dental Research*, 52:1041-1045.

[24] McNamara JA. (1973). Neuromuscular and skeletal adaptations to altered function in the orofacial region. *American Journal of Orthodontics*, 64:578.

[25] Milidonis MK, Kraus S. (1993). Genioglossi muscle activity in response to changes in anterior/neutral head posture. *American Journal of Orthodontics*, 103:39-44.

[26] Mohl ND. (1976). Head posture and its role in occlusion. NY State *Dental Journal*, 42:17-23.

[27] Mohlin B, Sagne S, Thilander B. (1978). The frequency of malocclusion and the craniofacial morphology in a medieval population in Southern Sweden. *Ossa*, 5:57-84.

[28] Murphy T. (1958). Mandibular adjustment to functional tooth attrition. *Australian Dental Journal*, 3(3):171-178.

[29] Preston CB, Evans WG, Rumbak A. (1996). An evaluation of two methods used to determine the centre of gravity of a cadaver head in the sagittal plane. *Journal of American Dental Assoc S Afr.* 51:787-793.

[30] Sakaguchi K, Mehta NR, Abdallah EF, et al. (2007). Examination of

the relationship between mandibular position and body posture. *Journal of Craniomandibular Practice*, 25(4):237-249.

[31] Schwartz AM. (1928). Positions of the head and malrelations of the jaws. *Int Journal of Orthod Oral Surgery Radiol*, 14:56-68.

[32] Solow B, Kreiborg S. (1977). Soft-tissue stretching: a possible control factor in craniofacial morphogenesis. *Scandinavian Journal of Dental Research*, 85:505-507.

[33] Solow B, Sonnesen L. (1998). Head posture and malocclusions. *European Journal of Orthodontics*, 20:685-693.

[34] Wentzel A, Williams S, Ritzau M. (1989). Changes in head posture and nasopharyngeal airway following surgical correction of mandibular prognathism. *European Journal of Orthodontics*, 11:37-42.

[35] Kibana Y, Ishijima T, Hirai T. (2002). Occlusal support and head posture. *Journal of Oral Rehabilitation*, 29(1):58-63.

[36] Katsaros C. (2001). Masticatory muscle function and transverse dentofacial growth. *Swedish Dental Journal Suppl*, 151:1-47.

[37] Menegaz, Rachel. (2010). "Craniofacial developmental instability and masticatory behavior [abstract]." *2009 Health Sciences Research Day (MU)*.

[38] Kiliaridis S. (2006). The importance of masticatory muscle function in dentofacial growth. *Seminars in Orthodontics*, 12(2):110-119.

[39] Gonzalez, H. E., & Manns, A. (1996). Forward Head Posture: Its Structural and Functional Influence on the Stomatognathic System, a Conceptual Study. *CRANIO®*, 14(1), 71-80.

[40] Huggare J. (1998). Postural disorders and dentofacial morphology. *Acta Odontologica Scandinavica*, 56(6):383-386.

[41] Solow B, Tallgren A. (1976). Head posture and craniofacial morphology. *American Journal of Physical Anthropology*, 44:417-436.

[42] Solow B, Tallgren A. (1977). Dentoalveolar morphology in relation to craniocervical posture. *The Angle Orthodontist*, 47:157-164.

[43] Ferrario VF, Sforza C, Serrao G. (1999). The influence of crossbite on the coordinated electromyographic activity of human masticatory muscles during mastication. *Journal of Oral Rehabilitation*, 26:575-581.

[44] Karlsson S, Ch SA, Carlsson GE. (1992). Changes in mandibular

masticatory movements after insertion of non working side interference. *Journal of Craniomandibular Disorder*, 6:177-183.

[45] Shimazaki T, Motoyoshi M, Hosoi K, Namura S. (2003). The effect of occlusal alteration and masticatory imbalance on the cervical spine. *European Journal of Orthodontics*, 25(5):457-463.

[46] Goldberg CJ , Moore DP, Fogarty EE, Dowling FE. (2002). The relationship between minor asymmetry and early idiopathic scoliosis. *Studies in Health Technology and Informatics*, 88:17-19.

[47] Sforze C, Tartaglia GM, Solimene U, Morgun V, et al. (2006). Occlusion, sternocleidomastoid muscle activity, and body sway: a pilot study in male astronauts. *Journal of Craniomandibular Practice*, 24(1):43-49.

[48] Rasmussen O C, Bonde-Petersen F, Christiensen L V, Moller E. (1977). Blood flow in human mandibular elevators at rest and during controlled biting. *Archives Oral Biology*, 22(8-9):539-43.

[49] Moller E, Rasmussen OC, Bonde-Petersen F. (1979) Mechanism of ischemic pain in human muscles of mastication: intramuscular pressure, EMG, force and blood flow of the temporal and masseter muscles during biting. *Advances in Pain Research and Therapy vol 3*. John Bonica et al. (eds) Raven Press, N.Y.

[50] Bonde-Petersen F, Christiensen LV. (1973). Blood flow in human temporal muscle during tooth grinding and clenching as measured by Xenon clearance. *Scandanavian Journal of Dental Research*, 81:272-275.

[51] Greenbaum, T., Dvir, Z., Reiter, S., & Winocur, E. (2017). Cervical flexion-rotation test and physiological range of motion – A comparative study of patients with myogenic temporomandibular disorder versus healthy subjects. *Musculoskeletal Science and Practice*, 27, 7–13.

[52] Goldstein, D. F., Kraus, S. L., Willams, W. B., & Glasheen-Wray, M. (1984). Influence of cervical posture on mandibular movement. *The Journal of Prosthetic Dentistry*, 52(3), 421–426.

[53] Milanesi JM et al. (2011). Impact of the mouth breathing occurred during childhood in the adult age: bio photogrammetric postural analysis. *Int. Journal of Pediatric Otorhinolaryngology*, Aug 75(8):999-1004.

[54] Krakauer L.H. and Guilherme A. (2000). Relationship between mouth breathing and postural alterations of children: a descriptive analysis. *Int. Journal of Orofacial Myology*, 25(1): 13-23.

[55] https://pdfs.semanticscholar.org/4338/43b8b1d85a18085de17e1ac29d148 3cb7ef8.pdf

[56] Scoppa, F., & Pirino, A. (2019). Is there a relationship between body posture and tongue posture? Glosso-Postural syndrome between myth and Reality. *Acta Medica Mediterranea*, 35, 1903.

[57] Machado Júnior, A. J., & Crespo, A. N. (2012). Postural evaluation in children with atypical swallowing: radiographic study. *Jornal Da Sociedade Brasileira de Fonoaudiologia*, 24(2), 125–129.

[58] Korbmacher, H. et al. 2005. Orofacial myofunctional disorders in children with asymmetry of the posture and locomotion apparatus. International Journal of Orofacial Myology, 31(1):26-38.

Chapter 6

[1] Cuccia, A. M., Caradonna, C., Caradonna, D., Anastasi, G., Milardi, D., Favaloro, A., … Cutroneo, G. (2013). The arterial blood supply of the temporomandibular joint: an anatomical study and clinical implications. *Imaging Science in Dentistry*, 43(1), 37.

[2] Neumann DA (2010) *Kinesiology of the Musculoskeletal System: Foundations for Physical Rehabilitation, ed 2*, St Louis: Mosby. Fig. 11.10. https://clinicalgate.com/kinesiology-of-mastication-and-ventilation/

[3] Benjamin, M., & Ralphs, J. R. (2004). Biology of Fibrocartilage Cells. *International Review of Cytology*, 1–45.

[4] Milam, S. B. (2005). Pathogenesis of degenerative temporomandibular joint arthritides. *Odontology*, 93(1), 7–15.

[5] Bergman AA, Heidger PM. (1996) *Histology*. Iowa City, IA: W.B. Saunders Company.

[6] Symons, N. B. B. (1965). A histochemical study of the secondary cartilage of the mandibular condyle in the rat. *Archives of Oral Biology*, 10(4), 579-IN3.

[7] Omar Abubaker, A., F. Raslan, W., & C. Sotereanos, G. (1993). Estrogen and progesterone receptors in temporomandibular joint discs of symptomatic and asymptomatic persons: A preliminary study. *Journal of Oral and Maxillofacial Surgery*, 51(10), 1096–1100.

The ALF Approach

[8] Milam, S. B., Aufdemorte, T. B., Sheridan, P. J., Triplett, R. G., Van Sickels, J. E., & Holt, G. R. (1987). Sexual dimorphism in the distribution of estrogen receptors in the temporomandibular joint complex of the baboon. *Oral Surgery, Oral Medicine, Oral Pathology*, 64(5), 527–532.

[9] Aufdemorte, T. B., Van Sickels, J. E., Dolwick, M. F., Sheridan, P. J., Holt, G. R., Aragon, S. B., & Gates, G. A. (1986). Estrogen receptors in the temporomandibular joint of the baboon (Papio cynocephalus): An autoradiographic study. *Oral Surgery, Oral Medicine, Oral Pathology*, 61(4), 307–314.

[10] Yamada, K., Nozawa-Inoue, K., Kawano, Y., Kohno, S., Amizuka, N., Iwanaga, T., & Maeda, T. (2003). Expression of estrogen receptor alpha(ER alpha) in the rat temporomandibular joint. *The Anatomical Record*, 274A(2), 934–941.

[11] Wang WHT, Chen C, Kapila S. (2006). Relaxin and estrogen receptor expression in TMJ and knee fibrocartilages. *Journal of Dental Research*. 85:0021. abstract.

[12] Milam, S. B., Aufdemorte, T. B., Sheridan, P. J., Triplett, R. G., Van Sickels, J. E., & Holt, G. R. (1987b). Sexual dimorphism in the distribution of estrogen receptors in the temporomandibular joint complex of the baboon. *Oral Surgery, Oral Medicine, Oral Pathology*, 64(5), 527–532.

[13] LeResche, L., Saunders, K., Von Korff, M. R., Barlow, W., & Dworkin, S. F. (1997). Use of exogenous hormones and risk of temporomandibular disorder pain. *Pain*, 69(1), 153–160.

[14] Meisler, J. G. (1999). Chronic Pain Conditions in Women. *Journal of Women's Health*, 8(3), 313–320.

[15] Landi, N., Lombardi, I., Manfredini, D., Casarosa, E., Biondi, K., Gabbanini, M., & Bosco, M. (2005). Sexual hormone serum levels and temporomandibular disorders. A preliminary study. *Gynecological Endocrinology*, 20(2), 99–103.

[16] Gunson, M. J., Arnett, G. W., Formby, B., Falzone, C., Mathur, R., & Alexander, C. (2009). Oral contraceptive pill use and abnormal menstrual cycles in women with severe condylar resorption: A case for low serum 17β-estradiol as a major factor in progressive condylar resorption. *American Journal of Orthodontics and Dentofacial Orthopedics*, 136(6), 772–779.

[17] Milani RS, de Periere DD, Micallef J-P. (1998) Relationship between dental occlusion and visual focusing. *Journal of Craniomandibular Practice*, 16(2):109-118.

[18] Bouvier M. (1988). Effects of age on the ability of the rat temporomandibular joint to respond to changing functional demands. *Journal of Dental Research.* 67, 1206–12.

[19] Ravosa, M. J., Kunwar, R., Stock, S. R., & Stack, M. S. (2007). Pushing the limit: masticatory stress and adaptive plasticity in mammalian craniomandibular joints. *Journal of Experimental Biology*, 210(4), 628–641.

[20] Kiliaridis, S., Thilander, B., Kjellberg, H., Topouzelis, N., & Zafiriadis, A. (1999). Effect of low masticatory function on condylar growth: A morphometric study in the rat. *American Journal of Orthodontics and Dentofacial Orthopedics*, 116(2), 121–125.

[21] Pirttiniemi, P., Kantomaa, T., Salo, L., & Tuominen, M. (1996). Effect of reduced articular function on deposition of type I and type II collagens in the mandibular condylar cartilage of the rat. *Archives of Oral Biology*, 41(1), 127–131.

[22] Milani, R. S., de Periere, D. D., & Micallef, J.-P. (1998). Relationship Between Dental Occlusion and Visual Focusing. *CRANIO®*, 16(2), 109–118.

[23] Pirttiniemi, P. (2004). Effect of decreased loading on the metabolic activity of the mandibular condylar cartilage in the rat. *The European Journal of Orthodontics*, 26(1), 1–5.

[24] Sato, I., Uneno, R., Miwa, Y., & Sunohara, M. (2006). Distribution of tenascin-C and tenascin-X, apoptotic and proliferating cells in postnatal soft-diet rat temporomandibular joint (TMJ). *Annals of Anatomy – Anatomischer Anzeiger*, 188(2), 127–136.

[25] Chen, J., Sorensen, K. P., Gupta, T., Kilts, T., Young, M., & Wadhwa, S. (2009). Altered functional loading causes differential effects in the subchondral bone and condylar cartilage in the temporomandibular joint from young mice. *Osteoarthritis and Cartilage*, 17(3), 354–361.

[26] Boever, J. A., & Keersmaekers, K. (1996). Trauma in patients with temporomandibular disorders: frequency and treatment outcome. *Journal of Oral Rehabilitation*, 23(2), 91–96.

[27] Carroll, L. J., Ferrari, R., & Cassidy, J. D. (2007). Reduced or painful jaw movement after collision-related injuries. *The Journal of the American Dental Association*, 138(1), 86–93.

[28] Salé, H., & Isberg, A. (2007). Delayed temporomandibular joint pain and dysfunction induced by whiplash trauma. *The Journal of the American Dental Association*, 138(8), 1084–1091.

[29] Dworkin, S. F., LeResche, L., DeRouen, T., & Von Korff, M. (1990). Assessing clinical signs of temporomandibular disorders: Reliability of clinical examiners. *The Journal of Prosthetic Dentistry*, 63(5), 574–579.

[30] Von Korff, M., Dworkin, S. F., Le Resche, L., & Kruger, A. (1988). An epidemiologic comparison of pain complaints. *Pain*, 32(2), 173–183.

[31] Solberg, W.K (1982).. Epidemiology, incidence, and prevalence of temporomandibular disorders: a review. *Presented at the President's Conference on the Examination, Diagnosis, and Management of Temporomandibular Disorders*; Chicago.

[32] Felson, D. T., & Nevitt, M. C. (1998). The effects of estrogen on osteoarthritis. *Current Opinion in Rheumatology*, 10(3), 269–272.

[33] Warren, M. P., & Fried, J. L. (2001). Temporomandibular Disorders and Hormones in Women. *Cells Tissues Organs*, 169(3), 187–192.

[34] Carlsson, G.E., LeResche, L. (1995). *Epidemiology of Temporomandibular Disorders*. Seattle: IASP Press.

[35] Milidonis, M. K., Kraus, S. L., Segal, R. L., & Widmer, C. G. (1993). Genioglossi muscle activity in response to changes in anterior/neutral head posture. *American Journal of Orthodontics and Dentofacial Orthopedics*, 103(1), 39–44.

[36] Marşan, G., Öztaş, E., Cura, N., Vasfi Kuvat, S., & Emekli, U. (2010). Changes in head posture and hyoid bone position in Turkish Class III patients after mandibular setback surgery. *Journal of Cranio-Maxillofacial Surgery*, 38(2), 113–121.

[37] Wenzel, A., Williams, S., & Ritzau, M. (1989). Changes in head posture and nasopharyngeal airway following surgical correction of mandibular prognathism. *European Journal of Orthodontics*, 11(1), 37–42.

[38] Murphy, T. (1958). Mandibular adjustment to functional tooth attrition. *Australian Dental Journal*, 3(3), 171–178.

[39] Helm, S., & Prydsö, U. (1979). Prevalence of malocclusion in medieval and modern Danes contrasted. *European Journal of Oral Sciences*, 87(2), 91–97.

[40] Mohlin, B., Sagne, S., Thilander, B. (1978). The frequency of malocclusion and the craniofacial morphology in a medieval population in Southern Sweden. *Ossa (International Journal of Skeletal Research)*, (5)57-84.

[41] Angel, J. L. (1976). Colonial to modern skeletal change in the U.S.A. *American Journal of Physical Anthropology*, 45(3), 723–735.

[42] Carlson, D. S., & Van Gerven, D. P. (1977). Masticatory function and post-pleistocene evolution in Nubia. *American Journal of Physical Anthropology*, 46(3), 495–506.

[43] Varrela, J. (1990). Occurrence of malocclusion in attritive environment: a study of a skull sample from southwest Finland. *European Journal of Oral Sciences*, 98(3), 242–247.

[44] Louveau, A., Smirnov, I., Keyes, T. J., Eccles, J. D., Rouhani, S. J., Peske, J. D., … Kipnis, J. (2015). Structural and functional features of central nervous system lymphatic vessels. *Nature*, 523(7560), 337–341.

[45] Crow, W. T., King, H. H., Patterson, R. M., & Giuliano, V. (2009). Assessment of calvarial structure motion by MRI. *Osteopathic Medicine and Primary Care*, 3(1), 8.

[46] Ueno, Toshiaki, et al. (1998) Noninvasive measurement of pulsatile intracranial pressure using ultrasound. *Intracranial Pressure and Neuromonitoring in Brain Injury*. Springer, Vienna. 66-69.

[47] Moskalenko, Y. E., Kravchenko, T. I., Gaidar, B. V., Vainshtein, G. B., Semernya, V. N., Maiorova, N. F., & Mitrofanov, V. F. (1999). Periodic mobility of cranial bones in humans. *Human Physiology*, 25(1), 51-58.

[48] Gardner, R. C., & Yaffe, K. (2015). Epidemiology of mild traumatic brain injury and neurodegenerative disease. *Molecular and Cellular Neuroscience*, 66, 75–80.

[49] Cruz-Haces, M., Tang, J., Acosta, G., Fernandez, J., & Shi, R. (2017). Pathological correlations between traumatic brain injury and chronic neurodegenerative diseases. *Translational Neurodegeneration*, 6(1).

[50] Graves, A. B., White, E., Koepsell, T. D., Reifler, B. V., Van Belle, G., Larson, E. B., & Raskind, M. (1990). The association between head trauma and Alzheimer's disease. *American Journal of Epidemiology*, 131(3), 491–501.

[51] Amor, S., Peferoen, L. A. N., Vogel, D. Y. S., Breur, M., van der Valk, P., Baker, D., & van Noort, J. M. (2014). Inflammation in neurodegenerative diseases – an update. *Immunology*, 142(2), 151–166.

[52] Eide, P. K., Vatnehol, S. A. S., Emblem, K. E., & Ringstad, G. (2018). Magnetic resonance imaging provides evidence of glymphatic drainage from human brain to cervical lymph nodes. *Scientific Reports*, 8(1).

[53] Plog, B. A., & Nedergaard, M. (2018). The Glymphatic System in Central Nervous System Health and Disease: Past, Present, and Future. Annual Review of Pathology: Mechanisms of Disease, 13(1), 379–394.

[54] Rasmussen, M. K., Mestre, H., & Nedergaard, M. (2018). The glymphatic pathway in neurological disorders. *The Lancet Neurology*, 17(11), 1016–1024.

[55] Isse, K., Kanamori, M., Uchiyama, M., Tanaka, K., Kuroda, A., Tanahashi, ... Kondo,K. (1991). A Case-Control Study of Risk Factors Associated with Alzheimer Type Dementia in Japan. In: Saytayoshi, E. (ed.) *Studies in Alzheimer's Disease: Epidemiology and Risk Factors Proceedings of the Third International Symposium on Dementia*. National Center of Neurology and Psychiatry. pp 63-67. Publishers, Tokyo.

[56] Andoh, T., Sakuma, Y., Yamamoto, S., Matsuno, A., Maeda, T., & Kotani, J. (2009). Influences of molar loss of rat on learning and memory. *Journal of Prosthodontic Research*, 53(4), 155–160.

[57] Miyamoto, M., Kato, J., Narumi, S., & Nagaoka, A. (1987). Characteristics of memory impairment following lesioning of the basal forebrain and medial septal nucleus in rats. *Brain Research*, 419(1–2), 19–31.

[58] Hwang, Y.K. & Chun, J.S. & Yoo, P.D. & Ma, J.Y. & Hyun, B.H. & Kim, S.U. & Chang, K.T. & Lee, Sang-Han. (2004). Occlusal reduction of unilateral molars influences change of stress-related hormones in rats. *Scandinavian Journal of Laboratory Animal Science*. 31. 73-77.

[59] Yamamoto, T., & Hirayama, A. (2001). Effects of soft-diet feeding on synaptic density in the hippocampus and parietal cortex of senescence-accelerated mice. *Brain Research*, 902(2), 255–263.

[60] Terasawa, H., Hirai, T., Ninomiya, T., Ikeda, Y., Ishijima, T., Yajima, T., Hamaue, N., Nagase, Y., Kang, Y., & Minami, M. (2002). Influence of tooth-loss and concomitant masticatory alterations on cholinergic neurons in rats: immunohistochemical and biochemical studies. *Neuroscience Research*, 43(4), 373–379.

[61] Kato, T., Takahashi, S., & Domon, T. (2015). Effects of a Liquid Diet on the Temporomandibular Joint of Growing Rats. *Medical Principles and Practice*, 24(3), 257–262.

[62] Sims, A. B., Stack, B. C., & Demerjian, G. G. (2012). Spasmodic Torticollis: The Dental Connection. *CRANIO®*, 30(3), 188–193.

[63] Siegel, J. M., Tomaszewski, K. S., & Wheeler, R. L. (1983). Behavioral organization of reticular formation: studies in the unrestrained cat. II. Cells related to facial movements. *Journal of Neurophysiology*, 50(3), 717–723.

[64] Stack, B., & Sims, A. (2009). The Relationship Between Posture and Equilibrium and the Auriculotemporal Nerve In Patients with Disturbed Gait and Balance. *CRANIO®*, 27(4), 248–260.

[65] Stack, B., & Sims, A. (2009b). The Relationship Between Posture and Equilibrium and the Auriculotemporal Nerve In Patients with Disturbed Gait and Balance. *CRANIO®*, 27(4), 248–260.

[66] Stack, B., & Sims, A. (2009c). The Relationship Between Posture and Equilibrium and the Auriculotemporal Nerve In Patients with Disturbed Gait and Balance. *CRANIO®*, 27(4), 248–260.

[67] Kendall, F. P., & McCreary, E. K. (1983). *Muscles: Testing and Function* (3rd ed.). Williams and Wilkins, Baltimore.

[68] Tripodakis, A. P., Smulow, J. B., Mehta, N. R., & Clark, R. E. (1995). Clinical study of location and reproducibility of three mandibular positions in relation to body posture and muscle function. *The Journal of Prosthetic Dentistry*, 73(2), 190–198.

[69] Pinganaud, G., Bourcier, F., Buisseret-Delmas, C., & Buisseret, P. (1999). Primary trigeminal afferents to the vestibular nuclei in the rat: existence of a collateral projection to the vestibulo-cerebellum. *Neuroscience Letters*, 264(1–3), 133–136.

[70] Darling, D. W., Kraus, S., & Glasheen-Wray, M. B. (1984). Relationship of head posture and the rest position of the mandible. *The Journal of Prosthetic Dentistry*, 52(1), 111–115.

[71] Bracco, P., Deregibus, A., & Piscetta, R. (2004). Effects of different jaw relations on postural stability in human subjects. *Neuroscience Letters*, 356(3), 228–230.

[72] Milani, R. S., De Perière, D. D., Lapeyre, L., & Pourreyron, L. (2000). Relationship Between Dental Occlusion and Posture. *CRANIO®*, 18(2), 127–134.

[73] https://www.ncbi.nlm.nih.gov/pmc/articles/PMC6780873/

[74] Bonaz B, Sinniger V, Pellissier S. Vagus nerve stimulation: a new promising therapeutic tool in inflammatory bowel disease. *J Intern Med* (2017) 282:46–63.

[75] Evrensel A, Ceylan ME. The gut-brain axis: the missing link in depression. *Clin Psychopharmacol Neurosci* (2015) 13:239–44.

[76] Leclercq S, Forsythe P, Bienenstock J. Posttraumatic stress disorder: does the gut microbiome hold the key? *Can J Psychiatry* (2016) 61:204–13.

[77] Goverse G, Stakenborg M, Matteoli G. The intestinal cholinergic anti-inflammatory pathway. *J Physiol* (2016) 594:5771–80.

[78] Berntson GG, Cacioppo JT, Quigley KS (March 1993). "Respiratory sinus arrhythmia: autonomic origins, physiological mechanisms, and psychophysiological implications." *Psychophysiology*. 30 (2): 183–96.

[79] Berntson GG, Cacioppo JT, Quigley KS (March 1993). "Respiratory sinus arrhythmia: autonomic origins, physiological mechanisms, and psychophysiological implications." *Psychophysiology*. 30(2): 183–96.

[80] Frymann, V., DO, FAAO (1997). The Expanding Osteopathic Concept, Development of Cranial Bones, p. 54

[81] https://www.ncbi.nlm.nih.gov/books/NBK230871/

[82] Rosenberg, S. (2017). *Accessing the Healing Power of the Vagus Nerve: Self-Help Exercises for Anxiety, Depression, Trauma, and Autism*. Berkeley, CA: North Atlantic Books, p.177

[83] Porges, S. W., Bazhenova, O. V., Bal, E., Carlson, N., Sorokin, Y., Heilman, K. J., … Lewis, G. F. (2014). Reducing Auditory Hypersensitivities in Autistic Spectrum Disorder: Preliminary Findings Evaluating the Listening Project Protocol. *Frontiers in Pediatrics*, (2)80.

[84] Eide, P. K., Vatnehol, S. A. S., Emblem, K. E., & Ringstad, G. (2018). Magnetic resonance imaging provides evidence of glymphatic drainage from human brain to cervical lymph nodes. *Scientific Reports*, 8(1).

[85] Iliff, J. J., Thrane, A. S., & Nedergaard, M. (2017). The Glymphatic System and Brain Interstitial Fluid Homeostasis. *Primer on Cerebrovascular Diseases*, 17–25.

[86] Porges, S. W. (2009). The polyvagal theory: New insights into adaptive reactions of the autonomic nervous system. *Cleveland Clinic Journal of Medicine*, 76(4 suppl 2), S86–S90.

[87] Porges, S. W. (2001). The polyvagal theory: phylogenetic substrates of a social nervous system. *International Journal of Psychophysiology*, 42(2), 123–146.

88 Van Der Kolk, B. (2014). *The body keeps the score: brain, mind, and body in the healing of trauma.* New York: Viking Penguin. p. 80. ISBN 9780670785933. Retrieved 3 February 2018.

89 Okşayan, R., Sökücü, O., & Üçüncü, N. (2015). The Effects of Low-Level Laser Therapy on Condylar Growth with a Mandibular Advancement Appliance in Rats. *Photomedicine and Laser Surgery,* 33(5), 252–257.

Chapter 7

1 Pottenger, F. (1983) *Pottenger's Cats.* Price-Pottenger Nutrition Foundation, Inc.

2 McKeown, P. (2003). *Close Your Mouth.*

3 Page, M. (1997) *Degeneration Regeneration.* International Foundation for Nutrition and Health. Original 1956 by The Page Foundation, Inc.

4 Kelley, W. http://www.drkelley.com/*CANLIVER55*.html

5 Nemechek, P. (2017) *The Nemechek Protocol for Autism and Developmental Disorders.* Autonomic Recovery LLC.

Credits and Permissions

Chapter 2

76	Illustration by Adam Knauer.
79	Illustration by Adam Knauer.
87	Illustration by Adam Knauer.
88	Illustrations by Adam Knauer.

Chapter 3

98   Reproduced with permission from Dr. Andrew Haltof, DO. Modified by Adam Knauer.

99   From the Merck Manual Consumer Version (Known as the Merck Manual in the US and Canada and the MSD Manual in the rest of the world), edited by Robert Porter. Copyright 2020 by Merck Sharp & Dohme Corp., a subsidiary of Merck & Co., Inc., Kenilworth, NJ. Available at

http://www.merckmanuals.com/consumer. Accessed 5/20/2020.

101   Reproduced with permission from Dr. Andrew Haltof, DO. Modified by Adam Knauer.

102 - upper   Reproduced with permission from Dr. Andrew Haltof, DO.

102 - lower   Illustration by Adam Knauer.

107   Netter medical illustration used with permission from Elsevier. All rights reserved. Modified by Adam Knauer.

109   Photo provided by Tasha Turzo, DO, with parental consent.

110   Photo provided by Tasha Turzo, DO, with parental consent.

Chapter 4

126   Photos provided by Kathy Winslow, BS, RDH, COM™ with parental consent.

127   Photos provided by Kathy Winslow, BS, RDH, COM™ with parental consent.

128   Photos provided by Kathy Winslow, BS, RDH, COM™ with parental consent.

134   Photo provided by Kathy Winslow, BS, RDH, COM™ with parental consent.

135 - upper   Jmarchn, CC BY-SA 3.0 <https://creativecommons.org/licenses/by-sa/3.0>, via Wikimedia Commons.

135 - middle Photos provided by Kathy Winslow, BS, RDH, COM™ with parental consent.

135 - lower   Photos provided by Kathy Winslow, BS, RDH, COM™ with parental consent.

Chapter 5

141	© SciePro / Adobe Stock.
142	Illustration by Adam Knauer.
143 - upper	Reproduced with permission from Fabio Scoppa.
	Scoppa, F., & Pirino, A. (2019). Is there a relationship between body posture and tongue posture? Glosso-Postural syndrome between myth and Reality. *Acta Medica Mediterranea*, 35, 1903.
143 - lower	Illustration by Adam Knauer.
146	Illustration by Adam Knauer.
148	© Marina / Adobe Stock.
149	Photo provided by Tasha Turzo, DO, with parental consent.
150	Illustration by Adam Knauer.
152 - upper	© Xavier / Adobe Stock.
152 - lower	Illustration by Adam Knauer.
157	Illustration by Adam Knauer.
158	Original source unknown. Modified by Adam Knauer.
161	Geof Sheppard, CC BY-SA 4.0 <https://creativecommons.org/licenses/by-sa/4.0>, via Wikimedia Commons. Modified by Adam Knauer.
162	Reproduced with permission from Tasha Turzo, DO. Modified by Adam Knauer.
163	Scoppa, F., & Pirino, A. (2019). Is there a relationship between body posture and tongue posture? Glosso-Postural syndrome between myth and Reality. *Acta Medica Mediterranea*, 35, 1903.

Chapter 6

167	Reproduced with permission from Dr. Andrew Haltof, DO.
170	Illustration by Adam Knauer.
177	Illustration by Adam Knauer.
181	Netter medical illustration used with permission from Elsevier. All rights reserved.
187	Netter medical illustration used with permission from Elsevier. All rights reserved.
188	Photo from 3D4Medical Complete Anatomy 2021 app.
189	Netter medical illustration used with permission from Elsevier. All rights reserved. Modified by Adam Knauer.
192	Netter medical illustration used with permission from Elsevier. All rights reserved.
194	Photo from 3D4Medical Complete Anatomy 2021 app.

Chapter 7

About the authors

Glossary

biocompatible: coexists with other living tissues without causing any harm

craniofacial cervical complex: bones and soft tissues of the face and the cranium

dental occlusion: the contact between teeth. More technically, it is the relationship between the maxillary and mandibular teeth when they approach each other, as occurs during chewing or at rest.

extra-oral: outside of the mouth

fascia: a band or sheet of connective tissue, primarily collagen, beneath the skin that attaches, stabilizes, encloses, and separates muscles and other internal organs.

fossa: an anatomical pit, groove, or depression

frenulum: (also called frenum) a small fold or ridge of tissue of the skin beneath the tongue, or between the lip and the gum.

glymphatic system: a functional waste clearance pathway for the vertebrate central nervous system.

hypoglossal nerve: the twelfth cranial nerve that innervates all the extrinsic and intrinsic muscles of the tongue, except for the palatoglossus, which is innervated by the vagus nerve. The hypoglossal nerve has solely a motor function. Basically, it's the nerve that moves the tongue.

intra-oral: inside the mouth

malocclusion: imperfect positioning of the teeth when the jaws are closed

mandible: the lower jawbone

maxilla: the upper jawbone. In humans it also forms part of the nose and eye socket.

musculoskeletal: relating to or denoting the musculature and skeleton together

orofacial myofunctional therapy: a program of specific exercises that target the facial muscles used to chew and swallow. These exercises strengthen the tongue as well as the muscle of chewing and swallowing.

neurodegenerative diseases: are debilitating conditions that result in progressive degeneration and/or death of nerve cells.

occipital condyle: each of two rounded knobs on the occipital bone that form a joint with the first cervical vertebra.

occiput: the back of the head or skull

oral myofunctional dysfunction: when there is an abnormal lip, jaw, or tongue position during rest, swallowing or speech. You may also see this when there are prolonged oral habits, like thumb or finger sucking.

orofacial dysphagia: refers to problems with using the mouth, lips and tongue to control food or liquid.

palate: the roof of the mouth in humans and other mammals. It separates the oral cavity from the nasal cavity.

sleep apnea: a potentially serious sleep disorder in which breathing repeatedly stops and starts.

somatic: relating to the body, especially as distinct from the mind

tongue thrust (also called reverse swallow or immature swallow): the common name of an oral myofunctional disorder, a dysfunctional muscle pattern in which the tongue protrudes anteriorly or laterally during swallowing, during speech, and while the tongue is at rest.

tongue-tie (ankyloglossia): a condition that restricts the tongue's range of motion. The condition is present at birth. A short, tight band of tissue tethers the tongue's tip to the floor of the mouth. It can affect how a child eats and speaks, and can interfere with breastfeeding.

torticollis: a condition in which the neck muscles contract, causing the head to twist to one side

vagus nerve: (also called cranial nerve X or cranial nerve 10) the longest and most complex of the cranial nerves. The vagus nerve runs from the brain through the face and thorax to the abdomen.

About the Authors

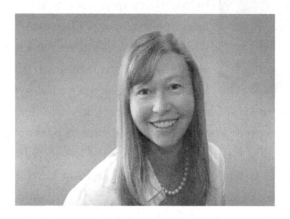

Dr. Tasha Turzo, DO, graduated from Western University, Pomona, California in 1994 where she received a Post Graduate Osteopathic Manual Medicine/Anatomy Fellowship. She completed her internship at the UCSF Family Medicine Residency. She has been in private practice since 1995 practicing osteopathy, homeopathy, functional medicine, prolotherapy/PRP and specializing in craniofacial dysfunctions. Dr. Turzo has been teaching extensively in the field of craniofacial dysfunctions since 1997. She began co-treating patients with Dr. Nordstrom (creator of the ALF appliances) in 1995. She is a founding member of AEI (ALF Educational Institute) and has taught (to date, 2021) 30 weekend courses to osteopaths, dentists and myofunctional therapists. Dr. Turzo has taught a 2-day online course "Osteopathy and the Dental Occlusion" twice a year since 2018. Dr. Turzo is an internationally recognized expert in the application of osteopathy and functional dentistry, with a focus on the use of the Advanced Lightwire Functional (ALF) devices and TMD. Dr. Turzo is also medical director of RevIVe Santa Cruz, a nutritional IV and injectables clinic. Her passions are transformational health, her daughters, and the love of her life, her husband.

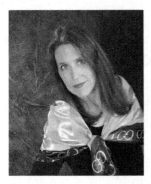

Kathy Winslow, BS, RDH, COM™, has been an Orofacial Myofunctional Therapist (OMFT) since 2004. She was raised in an "oral health-focused" environment as her father was an integrative dentist. His hygienist, Joy Moller, who is now a well-known educator in OMFT, was one of her first mentors. Kathy received her license as a registered dental hygiene in 1979 and has a BS in Oral Health. Kathy's curiosity and dedication to her clients and the profession have motivated her to pursue a broad range of advanced OFMT education. She is an IAOM-accredited COM™ as well as AOMT-trained. She is a Buteyko Educator Level 3, trained with MNRI (Facial Neuro-Reflex Integration), Haller Method, Lois Laynee, and has been on faculty for the ALF Educational Institute since 2014. She has been married 37 years to a handsome, surfing scientist who still makes her laugh!

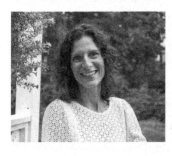

Traci Zimmerman Jones, DO, has a BS in Molecular Biology and is a 2004 graduate of Lake Erie College of Osteopathic Medicine. She is Board Certified in Family Medicine, completing her residency in Family Medicine at Dewitt Army Community Hospital, Fort Belvoir, VA in 2007. Her private practice, located in Centreville, VA since 2015, focuses on osteopathy and whole food nutrition. Dr. Jones has completed the AEI (ALF Educational Institute) Level 1 and 2 and currently works in collaboration with ALF dentists in the Washington, DC metro area treating craniofacial dysfunctions in patients of all ages. She is passionate about teaching parents and health care providers early intervention to optimize facial growth and development. She and her husband, Brian Jones, DO, have fully embraced the ALF approach while raising their two beautiful daughters.

Made in the USA
Middletown, DE
27 February 2025

71964389R00174